Winning at Losing

A Complete Program for Losing Weight and Keeping It Off

Rebecca Cavnar, R.N.

SERVANT BOOKS
Ann Arbor, Michigan

Cover photo by John B. Leidy © 1983 Servant Publications
Jacket and book design by John B. Leidy

Published by Servant Books
P.O. Box 8617
Ann Arbor, Michigan 48107

Printed in the United States of America
ISBN 0-89283-157-X

To Mother and Dad

Contents

Acknowledgments

THE AUTHOR GRATEFULLY acknowledges use of the following materials:

Eating Place Record from *Learning to Eat,* by James M. Ferguson, M.D., Bull Publishing Co., Palo Alto, CA 94302. Used with permission.

The food exchange lists in Appendix C are based on those prepared by committees of the American Diabetes Association, Inc., and The American Dietetic Association in cooperation with the National Institute of Arthritis, Metabolism and Digestive Diseases and the National Heart and Lung Institute, National Institutes of Health, Public Health Service, U.S. Department of Health, Education and Welfare. Copyright American Diabetes Association, Inc., The American Dietetic Association, 1976. These lists are also based on ones found in R.B. Stuart's and B. Davis' *Slim Chance in a Fat World* (Champaign, Illinois: Research Press Co., 1972) and are used with permission.

I would also like to thank Winslow G. Fox, M.D., for his support and encouragement in the beginning phases of my work in weight control; Daniel D. Heffernan, M.D., for continued support and patience with my work; Ellen H. Gryniewicz, M.D., for council and advice, especially concerning the particular needs of my women patients; and Ann Spangler, my hardworking editor, who helped pull this together.

Introduction

As far back as I can remember, I was overweight. I never knew why. I have four brothers and a sister, none of whom ever needed to lose weight.

I learned early in life to avoid eating very much in public. Instead, I ate when no one else was around. I hated the way I looked; it was always depressing to shop for clothes. My wardrobe was purchased in the "chubby girl" department.

Fortunately, I had loving and supportive parents who helped me develop many skills and interests. As a result, I was able to compensate for my weight problem. Academically and socially I managed to be a success.

Even so, I could not understand why I was fat and everyone else was thin. I never even liked fat people, so how could I be one of them? No one else seemed to understand why I was overweight either. The only advice I ever heard was "Just don't eat so much." But I had tried diets and failed. No matter how good my intentions or how "foolproof" the diet, I just could not take the weight off and keep it off. Though I knew that this area in my life was out of control, I did my best to deny it, to hide it, and to pretend it really was not a problem for me. Someday, I will lose weight, I reasoned. I just haven't really put my mind to it.

After I gave my life to the Lord, I put the idea aside for a while. It was clear to me that God had other priorities for my life just then. But in the back of my mind I began to expect that my weight problem would simply vanish once I matured enough as a Christian. As the years went by with no sign of that happening, I began to lose hope. If the Lord can't do it, who can? I asked myself. I reached an all-time high on the scales and an all-time low emotionally. Somehow, it never occurred to me that losing weight might require work on my part.

Finally, I began to tackle the problem head on. I began to diet. I decided to talk about my difficulty and to ask for support from others. And I began to have new hope, both for myself and for others in the same situation.

As a result of that hope, I have been able not only to lose weight and keep it off but to help others do the same. In order to successfully control a weight problem, certain tools are necessary. I have written this book in order to share with you some of the tools that I have found helpful. If you are serious about wanting to control your weight, I urge you to begin taking the necessary steps—to read, pray, and talk about it, and to get whatever help you need.

Another of my reasons for writing this book is to give you a straightforward, practical approach to weight loss. What is offered is much more than a diet. A diet will help you lose weight, but it won't help you keep it off. To really succeed, you will need a step-by-step program to help you recognize the factors in your daily life that contribute to your weight problem. Once you learn what these are, certain techniques will help you overcome each problem area. In essence, I hope to offer you a set of guidelines that will help you develop the kind of lifestyle which will enable you to control and manage your weight.

Unfortunately, many of the Christian books on the subject tend to overspiritualize the area, leaving the reader still overweight but now burdened with guilt. I am convinced that it takes a lot of hard work and perseverance to lose weight, but I do not think it is necessary to repent for every extra piece of bread you eat. God doesn't judge you by how well you are doing on your diet. What I want to offer you is not just a method to lose weight, but a way to become free of the guilt and self-condemnation that often plague Christians who are overweight.

Before we go any further, I would like to say a few things about how to support someone you love who is overweight.

Helping Someone Else Who Is Overweight

If your spouse, child, or best friend has a weight problem, the most helpful thing you can do is to love them as they are right now. If your love is based on their ability to lose weight, they will only experience pressure, anxiety, defeat, and possibly despair. You don't have to be glad that they are overweight. They are probably more distressed about the problem than you are. But if their weight is uppermost in your mind, your attitude will only place the kind of stress on the relationship that will cause them to eat more anyway. A pressured approach rarely succeeds. If this has been your attitude, let go of it. Ask God to show you how to love and accept the person as he is.

What if someone close to you does decide to lose weight? He is serious about it and asks for your support. What can you do? First of all, ask what kind of support he wants. He may be thinking of something very different than the kind of help you had in mind. He may ask you to take an active part to help him stay on his diet. Or he may prefer that you let him handle it unless he requests support in a specific situation. Some people appreciate a friend's efforts to stop them from eating a high-calorie food. They aren't offended when someone asks, "Is that on your diet?" or "Do you really want to eat that?" But others will be deeply offended by such questions. Some people want their friends to trust their determination and ability to stick to their diet.

If you want to support a person's efforts to lose weight, consider refraining from eating high-calorie food in his or her presence. This is similar to deciding not to drink in front of an alcoholic. Of course you probably cannot always avoid eating desserts and rich foods in front of people who are dieting, but you can be considerate, making adjustments where possible in a variety of situations. For instance, if your husband, who is on a diet, asks you out to dinner you can forgo dessert. Your small sacrifice will make life more pleasant for him.

As a general rule it is best to offer lots of encouragement and praise and very little, if any, correction or criticism. Usually overweight people have been corrected and criticized about their weight all their life. Receiving praise and encouragement from you could constitute a first for them. If you notice that someone took two rolls instead of one, ignore it. But if you notice that the person passed up dessert, praise him for it, either on the spot or a little later. But be sensitive. What one person perceives as encouragement another perceives as criticism. You may find that the overweight person is a bit touchy about the subject. Perhaps he is overly sensitive. Even so, you should do your best to consider how you can best support such a person.

Whatever you do, never try to bribe someone to lose weight. It will not work. The motivation and enthusiasm for losing weight must come from within. Your offer of a special gift or an exotic vacation may motivate the person for a while, but it probably will not carry him through the rough times. If the initiative does not come from the person himself, no amount of cajolery is likely to help. Such well-intentioned attempts often serve only to reinforce a sense of defeat.

Usually it is best if someone other than the husband or wife provides the primary support for the dieter. A spouse can find it difficult to remain objective while supervising a diet. It is easy to offer love and acceptance when the dieter is having a good day. But when the diet is not going so well, the husband or wife may take it personally, withdrawing a measure of love and acceptance when the other person needs it most. For that reason, it sometimes makes sense to go to a health professional or a weight-control group for guidance and support.

Children

Please do not blame the child for being fat. It isn't his fault. Of course something has caused the weight problem—the reason may be genetic or environmental—but it is not the child's fault, any more than it is to the thin child's credit that he is thin.

The overweight child may have a slow metabolism. He may

be less active, preferring to read or watch TV. He may have a fondness for sweets and rich foods. His body may not experience the sensation of "fullness." If that is the case, he will tend to eat large amounts of food before feeling full, if he ever feels full at all. He may become depressed and eat to console himself. Whatever the reason, do not blame the child. Some young children never even connect the act of eating with the size of their body.

Whatever the cause of the weight problem, the child does need your help. He needs a great deal of love, acceptance, praise, and encouragement. In fact, he probably needs more of these than the average child. The thin child may frequently hear comments such as, "Isn't she cute?" or "Isn't he handsome." The overweight child never receives such compliments. Perhaps he hears only, "My, isn't he big," or some such insensitive or cruel remark.

Never criticize or punish the child for being overweight. I know of an extreme case in which a father locked his son in his room for two or three days at a time to keep him away from food. The boy continued to gain weight and suffered a good deal of emotional damage in the process.

Whatever you do, never allow the child to give in to self-pity about this problem or any other. You need to help him keep perspective, to give him hope. If you give up, where will he turn?

Your overweight child does need your help. He cannot tackle the problem without you. Look for the right time to work on it with him. Perhaps other things need work before he can begin to lose weight. Pray about it. Be sensitive to the Holy Spirit. Ask the Lord where and when to start.

If the time is right and your child is ready to lose weight, remember that you will be his main support. Both of you need to be willing to embark on the diet. It will make significant demands on each of you. If the child is young, the parent should accompany him to the doctor, dietician, or weight-control group. And of course the mother will have to make sure that menu and meal preparation accommodate the diet.

It is most helpful if the family simply follows a diet similar to the child's. Desserts and other high-calorie foods should be kept at a minimum. As a rule, such foods should not be kept in the house. It is hard enough for a mature adult to resist them, much less a young child. Make it as easy on your child as possible by deciding ahead of time to remove any stumbling blocks from his path.

Teach the child to compensate for his weight problem. Help him to develop other skills or gifts to boost his self-confidence. Perhaps he has musical talent or is good with numbers. Help him make the most of whatever gifts he does have. He needs to succeed at something. The more self-confident he becomes, the easier it will be for him to lose the weight.

ONE

Who Has a Weight Problem?

THIS IS NOT just another book on dieting, a handy guide to teach you how to lose twenty pounds in ten days. I am not going to tell you that it is easy to lose weight and keep it off. Losing weight is a lot of hard work. I know because I have done it. I want to share with you some of the methods and insights I have learned to apply to myself and to my patients. My goal is to teach you how you can lose weight and keep it off.

Environment and Weight

How much you weigh may depend to a great degree on your social environment. A few years ago a study was conducted on the relationship between social class and thinness.[1] It found that upper class women tend to be the thinnest, middle class women less so, and lower class women the least so. Among religious denominations, Protestants were the thinnest, Catholics were less so, and Jews were least so. Among Protestants, Episcopalians were the thinnest, Presbyterians less so, followed by Methodists and finally Baptists. Thinness seems to be controlled to a remarkable degree by the social environment. But, however important social environment may be, it is certainly not the only factor in weight problems.

Three main phenomena contribute to weight problems in our culture. One is the overabundance of food and the ease of getting it. Another is the custom of using food as much more than a source of nutrition. The last is inactivity. As members of a highly technological society, we tend to be extremely inactive.

The first step in taking charge of your weight problem is to accept it. Maybe that surprises you. But no problem can be dealt with unless you face it squarely and accept the fact that it is your problem.

The second step is to accept the circumstances of your life. You happen to live in an affluent society and that means that you will have to deal with the particular obstacles which that presents. Someday our own country may experience a food shortage. Under extreme circumstances, perhaps nobody will have a weight problem. But for now you will need to learn how to handle abundance.

For most people, food represents more than just a source of nutrition. It offers a way to relax, to celebrate, to recreate, to comfort and console ourselves when we are depressed, to reward ourselves when we succeed. We use it to show love and to relieve anxiety and tension. Eating is something we do when we are bored; it also serves as the focal point for sharing and fellowship. No wonder some of us have a weight problem!

To regain control of your weight, you will need to learn to use food primarily as a means for meeting your nutritional needs. It is fuel for your body. That doesn't mean that you should never take pleasure in eating or that you should never use food for secondary purposes. But it does mean that it's wrong to center your life or your family's life around food.

Of course, not everyone sees things this way. The food industry would like you to buy food for every conceivable purpose and occasion. Food is packaged attractively and placed at your fingertips, so that it takes little or no effort to stock your cupboards with delicious homemade-tasting treats or rare delicacies. It is advertised relentlessly, subtly or not so subtly, in the attempt to convince you that your life will be happier if you eat this or serve your family that.

But the food industry is not the only factor that contributes to our weight problems. Modern technology is another culprit.

Because we live in the 1980s we drive cars instead of walking; we use machines to wash our dishes and our clothes; and we even have our trash compacted so that we only have to make one trip to the street for garbage pick-up. A phone in every room spares us the effort of walking fifteen feet to answer it. It's wonderful. Or is it? Our extreme inactivity leads to more and more weight problems.

All right. You understand these things. You know that you buy too much food and serve it for too many different occasions. You know you need to be more active physically. But you really wonder if there are not other reasons for your weight problem. Somewhere in the back of your mind is the notion that perhaps something may be wrong with you physically. Or you may think that some deep hurt has led to your weight problem. You may be right.

Physical and Spiritual Factors

Medical problems that cause weight gain are rare, but they do occur. If you have any reason to suspect that you have a medical problem, see your doctor. He or she may be able to reassure you that you are perfectly healthy, just overweight. But at least the question will be settled once and for all.

But what about spiritual factors? Though most weight problems have a definite spiritual aspect to them, we need to be careful not to overspiritualize them. A common train of thought among Christians runs like this: I have a weight problem because I was unhappy as a child and began turning to food for comfort. When the Lord heals my emotions, I will automatically lose weight. In the meantime, there is not much sense in trying.

Of course there is something to be said for this approach. It may be true that a person's unhappy childhood has contributed to their weight problem. And it probably is true that the Lord wants to heal those memories from the past. But it is also true that in order to lose weight, a person will eventually need to change his or her patterns of behavior and go on a diet. In many cases the actual cause of the problem was healed long ago but the old habits persist. Any change will require concerted effort.

Another attitude I sometimes encounter from Christians involves expecting a miracle. "I am praying and asking the Lord to take away my appetite so that I can lose weight." All the while the person prays this, he continues to eat whatever high-calorie food he pleases.

Certainly it is right to pray about your weight and to ask for the Lord's help, even for a miracle. But it is not usually the best approach to simply continue on your normal path until the miracle occurs. The Lord may want you to exert some effort. The best attitude is an aggressive, teachable, patient one. You can decide that you really want to lose the weight, that you are willing to learn everything you can, do whatever you need to, and change what needs changing. All the while, you can still ask God for that miracle. Sometimes the Lord chooses to perform real miracles for people who are overweight, but normally he works to guide and bless our efforts, to give us insight and revelation, and to provide us with strength and support through others.

Our weight problem may be our most deplorable weakness. And yet isn't it in weakness that the Lord can make us strong? Again and again our difficulty can bring us to our knees before him, so that we acknowledge our weakness and his strength. As surprising as it may sound, our ongoing struggle with weight can indeed be a blessing if we place it in the Lord's hands, letting him teach us patience and endurance and in that way allowing him to build our character.

Is It a Sin to Be Overweight?

Don't overspiritualize your weight problem. For many people overeating is a compulsive behavior which has its roots back in early childhood. Wrongdoing may be involved in overeating, but it is generally better not to think of your diet in terms of right and wrong.

A friend of mine was about five pounds too heavy and

resolved to lose the weight. But each day she ate one or two more pieces of bread than she should have. She felt guilty about every infraction, and the guiltier she felt, the more she ate. In her eyes, her lack of control was a sin. I told her that she was setting very high standards for herself, probably even higher than the Lord's standards for her. I recommended that she view her diet as a personal undertaking rather than a spiritual one. As soon as she did, she was free to receive the Lord's love. She no longer became utterly discouraged every time she ate an extra piece of bread. As a result she did better on her diet and eventually lost the weight.

You may not be to blame for your weight problem, but that does not excuse you from taking responsibility for it. Your weight problem probably cannot be traced to one isolated cause. More likely it results from a combination of causes, few or none of which are "your fault." To say this is not to say that you are incapable of doing anything about it. Regardless of how you acquired the problem, it is your problem now. It's up to you, and no one else, to take hold of it and figure out what you are going to do about it.

Why Me?

Perhaps you consider yourself a fairly strong Christian, someone with considerable responsibilities, all of which you handle well. Why, then, this problem with food?

Most of us learn to control our impulses at a fairly young age. We learn that we cannot have everything we see in the store because Mommy and Daddy will not buy all these things for us. We also learn that stealing is a serious offense. So we quickly silence the impulse in us that wants to own just about everything we see. Later, when we get older and begin to have sexual impulses, we learn we can only properly satisfy them in marriage. In the meantime, we learn to train and discipline such impulses. In fact, we learn that we cannot give in to most of our impulses. To do so may be too expensive, sinful, or simply unwise. But food is not that expensive; it is not immoral; and it is readily available. From the time we are very young, we satisfy most of our food impulses. We usually go right ahead and eat whatever appeals to us. The more this food impulse is reinforced, the more demanding it becomes. Many people are quite mature and well-controlled in just about every area except this one. Though fully grown, they have never gained control over their desires for food. Instead, their impulse is in control of them.

Is Thinness a Virtue?

Isn't there something fundamentally wrong, you may wonder, if food still presents so much difficulty for you? Our culture esteems thinness. The thin person is often admired and held up as the model of integrity and personal success. To be thin is to be "together." It is easy to label yourself a failure no matter how successful, mature, or capable you may be, if you are overweight. This attitude especially characterizes women. It is socially acceptable for a man to be on the heavy side. But a large woman is thought to be unattractive and careless about her appearance.

How many times have people said to you after you have lost a few pounds, "You look great. You've lost a little weight, haven't you?" No one minds a compliment, but such a remark does imply that you would not have received the compliment if you had not lost the weight. People assume that being overweight indicates that something is wrong. They wonder why you have "let yourself go." But, in fact, nothing may be wrong. You may be doing just fine. Sometimes subtle comments like these can make it easy for you to exaggerate your own weight problem.

One of my patients was about fifteen pounds overweight. She was married to a very thin man, who was constantly pressuring her to lose weight. Even his family pressured her. Clearly, they placed a very high value on thinness. But their attitude only added unnecessary tension and unhappiness to their marriage. It did nothing to help the woman lose weight.

On more than one occasion people have asked me to help them lose weight that they did not need to lose. Here again, the pressure to be thin was so great that they imagined that they had a weight problem. If you are a thirty-five-year-old mother of three, you aren't going to weigh the same as when you were sixteen, and you don't need to. Set a realistic goal for yourself. If you look good and feel good wearing a size 10 or 12, there is no reason to try to fit into a size 6. If you have unrealistic expectations, let go of them. Try to set more realistic goals so that you can live up to the Lord's standards, rather than the world's.

Should I Diet with My Spouse?

Very often, difficulties develop when a husband and wife diet together. It can work, but beware of the problems.

Men can usually lose weight twice as fast as women though they have the same relative calorie restriction. Their bodies are more muscular and require more calories to keep going. Women's bodies have a higher percentage of fat. God designed them that way. But as a result, it usually takes a woman longer to lose weight than a man.

In addition, women are usually around food more than men. They have to think about it, buy it, prepare it, serve meals, and put away the leftovers. All of these occasions constitute opportunities to eat. It is possible to learn how to handle these temptations, but it certainly makes life more difficult than if you did not have the constant food reminders in the first place.

A woman's hormones also affect her weight. Because of hormonal shifts at different times of the month, a woman may retain fluid. Even if she sticks to her diet one week, her efforts might not show up on the scale until the following week.

Should you diet with your spouse? Only if you both find it supportive, and if you understand that you will not lose weight at the same rate. Whatever you do, don't compete with one another.

Resentment Doesn't Help

It does not help to be resentful about your weight problem. You must accept it and decide to change it. Let go of the resentment. Put aside the self-pity. Forgive your parents or your grandparents—anyone you might feel resentful towards, even the Lord. You will not be able to make any progress until you accept the problem as *your* problem. Once you do, you can start to take charge of it.

Consider the case of a child born with a crippled leg. He could deal with his problem in one of two ways. He could be resentful about it, not lifting a finger to help himself. In this case his family would have to wait on him for everything. He could even pray daily, asking the Lord to heal his leg, but still clinging to his resentment. Or he could take a totally different approach, deciding to embrace the handicap and make the best of it. He could make up his mind to excel in those areas where he does possess gifts. Most of us can guess which approach would get him the farthest.

The same principle is at work with a weight problem, in fact, with any problem. There is nothing wrong with disliking the fact that you have a weight problem. You don't have to love it. But you do have to accept it and decide that you are going to learn to do whatever is necessary to take charge of it.

Know Your Strengths and Weaknesses

It is important to understand the concept of willpower. Most people think of willpower as the ability to sit in front of a hot fudge sundae and say, through gritted teeth, "No, thank you, I don't care for any." That is a misconception. Willpower is the ability to know your strengths and weaknesses and to know how to work within them.

Consider the case of an alcoholic who has decided to stop drinking. If he were to keep a well-stocked liquor cabinet and to surround himself with friends who drank constantly, he would be courting disaster. Such behavior would be a mark of stupidity rather than strength. On the other hand, he would be exercising strength of will if he were to keep his home free from liquor and refuse to frequent bars with his friends. Such behavior would indicate that the alcoholic knew his weakness and how to overcome it.

It is the same with food. It is foolish to think that we can surround ourselves with high-calorie treats and resist the temptation to eat them. The person with willpower uses foresight, self-knowledge, and planning to prevent being confronted by irresistible and undesirable choices. This principle applies to any kind of temptation. Christians throughout the ages—including St. Paul, St. Augustine, and Thomas Aquinas—taught that to avoid sin one must avoid the occasion for sin.

Why Lose Weight?

Have you ever asked yourself why you want to lose weight? It can be enlightening to pose the question: How will being slim affect me? What do I think it will do for me?

It is important to be realistic about it. Losing weight *will* do some things for you. But there are many things it will not do. There are no guaranteed outcomes.

Losing weight will usually make you feel healthier. It will also make you feel better about yourself. More control over food and over your own impulses can be a great boost to your self-confidence. And that self-confidence usually affects other areas of your life. You will probably be more confident socially, with the result that people will respond to you more positively, partly because you are more attractive, but primarily because you are more confident.

Even so, losing weight is not going to solve all your problems. You will not necessarily find a spouse just because you are thinner, though your chances may be better. Neither will you be guaranteed that promotion at work just because you lose weight. Losing weight is not the answer to all of life's problems, though the overweight person can be tempted to think it is. But it can help you get a little closer to many of the things you want in life. If nothing else, it eliminates your scapegoat, so that you can face the real problem instead of blaming it on the "fat."

One of my patients, who was about fifteen pounds over-weight, was convinced that people disliked her because she was heavy. She lost the weight but felt that people still did not like her. But now she could no longer blame her weight. She began to understand that the way she related to people was governed by the assumption that they disliked her. She would seldom initiate a conversation or say hello if someone walked into the room. She simply assumed that they disliked her and would not want to talk to her. Once she recognized the problem, she decided that she should start assuming either that people did like her or that they were at least neutral. As a result, she began to take more initiative. The response of others was encouraging, and she began to realize that people in fact did like her. Getting rid of the extra weight got rid of her scapegoat and enabled her to face the real problem.

It is not necessary to wait to tackle your weight problem until all your expectations and motives are flawlessly perfect. Few of us would ever start. You may know that some of your motives are not quite what they should be. Ask the Lord to purify them and to help you to have realistic expectations about losing weight. Your motives can be transformed in the weight-losing process itself.

The Best Time to Start

There is definitely a right time to start. That right time may simply be the day you make up your mind to lose the extra weight. Or it may be a day when you bring your difficulty to the Lord and place it in his care. Perhaps he has shown you a particular course of action. Or he may lead you to a book, like this one, or to a particular person or class in order to provide you with guidance and support.

It is usually best to start when you are not experiencing a lot of stress in your life, when things are relatively stable and peaceful and you are able to devote time and energy to the effort. If this is a very busy, pressured season in your life, it is probably not a good time to try to lose weight. It does take time. You need to think, pray, read, and talk about it.

Before you decide to diet, take these three steps:

1. Ask yourself whether your life is in good order. Do you
   -have regular time for prayer?
   -have a regular daily schedule?
   -have good relationships with those around you, especially your spouse, or those you live with?
   -keep your commitments to
     -work?
     -service?
     -family responsibilities?

These areas do not have to be in perfect shape, but you should at least be working on them.

2. Pray about it. Is this the Lord's priority right now for your life? If you can say yes to the first question and it this seems the right time to lose weight, then it probably is the Lord's time, too.

3. Discuss it with someone you respect. Talk to someone whose opinion you value. Do they have any advice to offer you? They may be able to give you objective input that will help you make a wise decision.

If these three considerations support your decision to diet, then it probably is the right time for you. If you come up with a "no" to one of the steps, then you should reconsider. It may be better to wait until another time.

If you do decide to diet, it helps to start on the right day. It is best to begin on a Monday, at the beginning of a season. When I say season, I am not talking about weather but about the seasons of your life. If September is traditionally a time for starting new projects because that's when the kids go back to school, it might be good to wait until then. If it is two days before Christmas, it would be better to wait until January 2nd to get started.

Dealing with Defeat

What happens if you decide to go on a diet and you meet with one defeat after another, gaining rather than losing weight? Try leaving the diet for a while. If you remain on it and continue to experience defeat, you will only conclude that your efforts are doomed to failure, which is not true. More likely, it just is not the right time for you to be working on this area. Put it aside until the Lord shows you that it is time to tackle the problem again.

Sharon came to me shortly after she became a Christian. At 250 pounds, she knew that she had to lose weight and wanted to get started immediately. But after talking to her, I concluded that God probably wanted to do other things in her life first. She needed to find a good job and to begin strengthening her relationship with the Lord and with other Christians. Moreover, her self-image needed to be restored before she could expect to make significant progress on a diet.

When I mentioned my thoughts to her, she listened with great relief. She had simply assumed that it was her duty to lose weight quickly since being so overweight was not a good Christian witness. She was glad to let the Lord work in other areas before tackling this one.

A year later she returned and succeeded in losing the extra weight. The peace and order that were already established in her life made the process much easier.

The First Step

Enough warnings. If you have decided that it is time to lose weight, what comes next?

Whenever you try to change a behavior, it is important to identify the current patterns of that behavior. If you want to stop biting your fingernails, it would help if you knew some things about your habit—when do you usually do it? where are you? who is around? how are you feeling? and so on.

Your first assignment is to keep a record of your eating behavior. Eat as you normally would. Don't start your diet yet. That should wait until next week. This week keep what I call a food and behavior diary. You can use the pages at the back of the book for this week's diary, but you will want to purchase a notebook that can be conveniently carried wherever you go since you will be using it during the whole program. Each day's record will be contained on a separate page since the information will change from day to day.

Record each eating episode in your food and behavior diary immediately after you eat. If you wait, you will probably forget some of the information. Figure 1 offers an example of how your diary should look. Every time you eat, you should record the time, where you are, what you are doing, how you are feeling, who you are with, the degree of your hunger, and what you are eating. At first this may seem like a lot of work. But, believe me, this diary is immensely helpful, and it takes only a little time to keep it up.

The mere act of keeping the diary will change your eating behavior somewhat. Right now most of your eating is probably very spontaneous. Once you start observing yourself, it will become much less spontaneous. The food and behavior diary will make you think before you eat something on an impulse. It is a little like trying to count how many times you breathe in a minute. Breathing is an automatic phenomenon. As soon as you start observing it, it ceases to be automatic and, therefore, changes. The same thing will happen when you begin to keep your diary.

This first week do your best to eat as you normally would. If you usually nibble on a piece of cheese while you are making lunch, then keep nibbling, just be sure to write it down.

After you have kept your diary for a week, review it. What patterns do you see? Where do you usually eat—standing up in the kitchen, driving in the car, or sitting at the dining room table? What do you do while you eat—watch TV, work at your desk, get together with friends? Do you tend to overeat when you are depressed or angry? Do you seem to eat more when you are alone than with others? Does your hunger seem related to how much you eat, or do you eat when you are not the least bit hungry?

The patterns you have observed this week will be of help as you begin to change your eating behavior. Save this initial food and behavior diary and refer back to it as you proceed to work on the behaviors one by one.

Week One Assignment:

Keep a food and behavior diary. This week, use the blank diary pages in Appendix A.

Figure 1
Food Diary Sample

Date ___Oct. 11___

Time	Place	Activity	Feeling	With Whom	Hunger	Food
7:30 A.M.	kitchen	watching the news	tired	alone	moderate	corn flakes milk orange juice coffee
10:20 A.M.	living room	visiting with neighbor	glad for a break	Jane	low	coffee cake butter coffee

TWO

Why Diet?

M OST OF US do not really know how to eat to stay thin. If we did, we probably would not be overweight. It is important to be on a balanced diet while you are losing weight, and it is crucial to *stay* on a balanced diet to *maintain* your weight. While losing weight, you can be learning a way to eat that will help you the rest of your life. But before starting this or any diet be sure to check with your doctor.

It helps to remember that the most fattening thing you can eat is fat. If people understood this, their attempts to lose weight might be more successful. I have often heard someone say, "I'm trying to lose weight, so no jelly on my toast, please." Then they proceed to spread butter or margarine on it. One teaspoon of butter or margarine has the same number of calories as three teaspoons of jelly!

Recently I was at a dinner party where some homemade biscuits were served. The woman next to me turned them down with regrets because she was watching her weight. Then she proceeded to place a one-inch slice of butter squarely on top of her green beans. It was unfortunate. The butter contained many more calories than one of the small biscuits. She simply did not realize what she was doing. The butter looks so small and the toast, biscuit, or potato looks so big. But butter, or any other kind of fat, is extremely dense in calories and therefore very fattening.

We like fat. It can make food taste better. That rich cake everyone loves has three sticks of butter in it. Fat is often a hidden source of calories—salad dressing, the mayonnaise in your tuna salad, butter on the vegetables, the oil used to fry foods, the fat on your pork chop. It seems so small, so harmless. But it really is a hidden villain. In fact, it is the most fattening thing you can eat.

Let's consider the main elements of a balanced diet. A sound diet consists of proportionate amounts of protein, carbohydrates, fats, vitamins, and minerals. Protein is needed for growth, metabolism, and the healing and upkeep of our bodies. The basic sources of protein are meats, poultry, fish, dairy products, beans, and seeds.

Carbohydrates supply sugar as fuel for the brain and muscle tissue. The sources of carbohydrates are starches, vegetables, and sugar. Any excess of protein or carbohydrate is converted to fat by our bodies.

Fats are simply a source of fuel storage. They are very high in calories. The sources of fats are mainly butter, margarine, oil, shortening, mayonnaise, and bacon. A weight-reduction diet should be relatively high in protein, moderate in carbohydrate, and quite low in fat.

"Vitamin" is a general term for a number of different organic substances that occur in many foods in small amounts. These substances are necessary for the normal metabolic functioning of the body. A deficiency of specific vitamins can cause disease. Vitamins are either water soluble or fat soluble.

Minerals are inorganic elements that play a vital role in metabolism. Sources of minerals include dairy products, vegetables, whole grains, meats, nuts, seeds, salt, and water. Appropriate amounts of all the minerals are essential to a balanced diet.

The ideal diet for both weight loss and weight maintenance provides sufficient amounts of all these essential dietary elements. The exchange diet, which I will explain below, is a simple, effective way to achieve this kind of balance.

Calories—How Many Do I Need?

Our calorie requirement can vary greatly at different times in our lives. A nineteen-year-old college football player can have a huge calorie requirement. The same man at age forty-five, with a sedentary desk job, would have a much lower calorie requirement. If he continues to eat anywhere near the amount that he did in college, he will certainly be overweight.

As you get older, your calorie requirement gradually drops. A forty-year-old woman and a five-year-old child have approximately the same calorie requirements. If you continue to eat the same way at fifty that you did at twenty-five, you will probably be overweight.

Occasionally I will see men or women in their early thirties who have developed a weight problem for the first time in their lives. They explain that they eat no differently than they ever have. Their weight gain is due in large part to their age but also to the fact that their activity level is lower than it was when they were younger. If they want to lose weight and keep it off, they will have to decrease their calorie intake.

For those who want to lose weight, I usually recommend 1,000 calories per day for women over thirty, 1,200 calories per day for women under thirty, and 1,500 calories per day for men or teenagers. These calorie recommendations are designed for people who get moderate exercise. You may choose more or less calories depending on the amount of exercise you get. Once you reach your goal weight, you can add calories daily until you reach the amount that will maintain your weight. Refer to Appendix B to determine how many calories are contained in particular kinds of food.

The Exchange Diet

In this diet, all foods are classified in seven groups: *meats, milks, breads, vegetables, fruits, fats or sweets,* and *free foods.* The foods within each group have approximately the same value in terms of nutrients and calories. One choice from any group is called an exchange. The diet which follows will tell you how many choices or "exchanges" you can have from each group in one day. For example, you might see that on the 1,000 calorie diet you can have three bread exchanges in a day. You could simply choose three pieces of bread. Or you could choose one ounce of breakfast cereal, five saltines at lunch, and a small baked potato at dinner. Each of these "starches" would be considered one bread exchange.

You can arrange the exchanges however you like, provided you have at least three meals. You must have at least breakfast, lunch, and dinner. If you like, you may use some of your exchanges for snacks.

Refer to Appendix C for the Food Exchange Lists. Notice that the top of each page lists how many calories are in one choice from that list. For instance, a fruit exchange equals approximately forty calories, whereas a milk exchange equals approximately eight-five calories. Free foods are those on the first page of the list. "Free" means that you can eat these foods whenever and in whatever quantity you desire. They do not need to be weighed or measured.

Choose the meal plan with the number of calories appropriate for you, and it will tell you the number of exchanges from each group that you may have in a day. You will also find a suggested breakdown of the exchanges throughout the day and a sample menu for one day. You may use this plan or develop your own. But be sure to use all the exchanges you are allowed.

1,000 Calorie Plan

Group	Number of Exchanges for One Day
meats	six
breads	three
milk (skim)	one
raw vegetables	free

cooked vegetables	three
fruit	three
miscellaneous	two

Suggested Menu Breakdown for One Day	**Sample Menu for 1,000 Calorie Diet**

Breakfast

Breakfast

1 bread exchange	1 oz. puffed rice
1 milk exchange	1 cup skim milk
1 fruit exchange	½ grapefruit
	1 tsp. sugar (part of a miscellaneous exchange)
	1 cup coffee, black

Lunch

Lunch

2 meat exchanges	cottage cheese
1 bread exchange	5 crackers
1 fruit exchange	1 small apple
1 cooked vegetable exchange	½ cup asparagus
raw vegetables as desired	lettuce salad with cucumber and tomato slices
½ miscellaneous exchange	low-calorie salad dressing (20 calories)
	tea, black

Dinner

Dinner

4 meat exchanges	4 oz. broiled flank steak
1 bread exchange	small baked potato
1 fruit exchange	pear
2 cooked vegetable exchanges	green beans steamed carrots
raw vegetables as desired	shredded cabbage salad

½ miscellaneous exchange

low-calorie dressing (20 calories)

½ tsp. butter

1,200 Calorie Plan

Group	Number of Exchanges for One Day
meats	six
breads	four
milks (skim)	two
raw vegetables	free
cooked vegetables	three
fruit	three
miscellaneous	three

Suggested Menu Breakdown for One Day

Breakfast

1 bread exchange
1 milk exchange
1 fruit exchange
1 miscellaneous exchange

Lunch

2 meat exchanges
1 bread exchange
1 fruit exchange
1 cooked vegetable exchange
raw vegetables as desired
½ miscellaneous exchange

Sample Menu for 1,200 Calorie Diet

Breakfast

1 oz. corn flakes
1 cup skim milk
½ cup orange juice
1 tsp. sugar
1 cup coffee, black

Lunch

2 oz. cheese
5 saltines
1 small apple
½ cup sauerkraut
lettuce salad
low-calorie salad dressing (20 calories)
tea, black

Snack	Snack
1 fruit exchange	pear

Dinner	*Dinner*
4 meat exchanges	4 oz. chicken
2 bread exchanges	½ cup rice
	dinner roll
2 cooked vegetable exchanges	1 cup broccoli
raw vegetables—as desired	lettuce salad with tomato and cucumber
1½ miscellaneous exchanges	low-calorie dressing (20 calories)
	1 tsp. butter
1 fruit exchange	1 cup strawberries
1 milk exchange	1/3 cup ice milk

1,500 Calorie Plan

Group	*Number of Exchanges for One Day*
meats	seven
breads	five
milk (skim)	two
raw vegetables	free
cooked vegetables	three
fruit	five
miscellaneous	five

Suggested Menu Breakdown for One Day	**Sample Menu for 1,500 Calorie Diet**
Breakfast	*Breakfast*
2 bread exchanges	2 oz. wheat flakes
1 milk exchange	1 cup skim milk
1 fruit exchange	½ cup orange juice

½ miscellaneous exchange

1 tsp. sugar
coffee, black

Lunch

3 meat exchanges

1 bread exchange
1 fruit exchange
1 cooked vegetable exchange
raw vegetables as desired
2 miscellaneous exchanges

Lunch

2 oz. tuna
1 hard-boiled egg
1 small roll
¼ cantaloupe
2 large stalks steamed broccoli
lettuce, celery, onion salad
1 tsp. mayonnaise
1 tsp. butter

Snack

1 fruit exchange

Snack

1 small apple

Dinner

4 meat exchanges
2 bread exchanges

2 cooked vegetable exchanges

raw vegetables as desired
1½ miscellaneous exchanges

1 fruit exchange &
1 milk exchange

Dinner

4 oz. baked chicken
½ cup cooked rice
1 small dinner roll
1 cup green beans
½ cup steamed carrots
sliced tomatoes
1 tsp. butter
1 tsp. salad oil with vinegar
banana milk shake (½ banana,
1 cup skim milk)

Snack

1 fruit exchange

Snack

1 orange

Some Helpful Hints

Be patient. If you have never used an exchange diet, you should not expect it to work overnight. It takes patience and practice, but it will soon seem like second nature.

In the beginning, *always* weigh and measure your foods. You may think you know what four ounces of steak looks like, but go ahead and weigh it (after it has been cooked). You may be surprised. I remember the first time I measured a teaspoon of mayonnaise. I simply could not believe it. "Is that all?" I wondered just how much I had been putting in my tuna salad. It probably should have been called mayonnaise salad.

Weigh and measure for at least the first three weeks, and then you can approximate. But if you are not sure, get the scale or the measuring spoons out again. You can consume a lot of extra calories if you overestimate.

Try to eat everything you plan to at a given meal. If you really do not want to finish your rice at dinner, that is fine. But don't try to cut back in order to lose weight faster. It will only set you up for trouble. If you eat everything you are supposed to eat at dinner, there is less chance that you will be hungry or feel deprived later on.

Make your diet fun and pleasant. You need not punish yourself because you are overweight. Make meals as tasty and pleasant as possible. Remember, what you eat at mealtime is all you are going to have (unless you plan a snack). You are not free to eat a candy bar in the afternoon because you only had an apple for lunch. It helps to plan meals that are both filling and appealing.

One pound of fat equals 3,500 calories. So, to lose a pound you need to reduce your calorie intake by 3,500 calories. A reduction of 500 calories a day or 3,500 calories a week would give you a weight loss of one pound per week. A reduction of 1,000 calories per day would mean a loss of two pounds a week.

More Hints

—Use a non-stick pan for browning and sauteing foods. It needs no grease at all. You can cook eggs or saute onions and mushrooms with a bit of water or boullion.

—Very thin-sliced breads or special low-calorie breads can

help you stretch your bread exchanges. Two slices of these usually equals only one bread exchange.

—Low-calorie dressings can save many calories. Read the label to see how many calories are in each tablespoon. Then count it accordingly as all or part of a miscellaneous exchange.

—Low-calorie hot cocoa and milk-shake mixes are tasty ways to use your milk exchanges. One serving of any of these can usually be counted as one milk exchange. Be sure to check the label. As long as a serving is under eighty-five calories, you may use it as a milk exchange.

—Low-calorie ice creams and frozen desserts are another way to use milk exchanges. Again, check the calorie amount on the carton.

—When browning meats, especially hamburger, pour it into a colander after browning well. This will drain off every possible drop of fat.

—Diet margarine will help stretch your miscellaneous exchanges. You can use two teaspoons for one miscellaneous exchange.

—Use skim milk to make mayonnaise go further in salads.

One Step at a Time

When you diet, take it one step at a time. If you look at the whole picture, it is easy to be overwhelmed. Don't say to yourself, "I can never eat a candy bar again." Instead, say, "Today I am not going to eat a candy bar." In fact, you really only need to think about the next hour. You can make it through the next hour, and that is all that is important. You need not worry about tonight, tomorrow, this weekend, Christmas, or the rest of your life. The Lord is giving you grace for the very next hour, and that is sufficient. After that hour is over, you can think about the next.

Use the chart at the end of this chapter to help you take it one step at a time this week. Down the left side of the chart, mark the hours of the day, starting with the earliest time you might get up. Now, for each hour that you stick to your diet, color in the box. If you eat something you should not be eating during a particular hour, leave it blank. But if the next hour goes well, color that hour in. For example, if you eat everything you are supposed to for breakfast, color in that hour. If you have a cup of coffee and an apple at 11:00 in accordance with your diet plan, then color in that hour.

Take it hour by hour. Your goal is to be able to color in the whole day, and then the whole week. If you go off your diet one hour, that's okay. Just get right back on it the next hour.

Don't Drown in Water You Can Stand Up In

Many people drown in water that they can actually stand up in. They panic and never even try to stand. Many times we do that when it comes to dieting. We panic and do not even try to stand up.

Next time you get into a difficult situation, don't panic. Tell yourself, "I will at least try. Maybe I can make it. Maybe I can do it. I'm not sure, but I will try." Chances are that you will succeed.

Rules to Remember

1. Never skip a meal.
2. Buy a food scale or postage scale to weigh any foods that need to be weighed.
3. Use measuring cups and measuring spoons to measure food.
4. Weigh in on the same day and at the same time each week. Do not weigh yourself at any other time.

Week Two Assignment:

1. Choose the diet plan that suits you. Read through the exchange lists, the suggested daily menu breakdown, and the sample menu.
2. Keep a simple food diary this week, using figure 2 as an example. This will be much easier than the detailed

diary you kept last week. Write down everything you eat as soon as you are done eating. Check off your exchanges on the checklist as you go through the day. That way you will know exactly how many you have left as you go along.

3. Fill out the hourly success chart, figure 3.

Figure 2-A
Food Diary for 1000 Calorie Diet

Date _____

Time   What I Ate

Meat
Bread
Cooked Veg.
Fruit
Misc.
Milk

Date _____

Time   What I Ate

Meat
Bread
Cooked Veg.
Fruit
Misc.
Milk

Date _____

Time   What I Ate

Meat
Bread
Cooked Veg.
Fruit
Misc.
Milk

Date _____

Time   What I Ate

Meat
Bread
Cooked Veg.
Fruit
Misc.
Milk

Figure 2-B
Food Diary for 1200 Calorie Diet

Date _____

Time   What I Ate

Meat
Bread
Cooked Veg.
Fruit
Misc.
Milk

Date _____

Time   What I Ate

Meat
Bread
Cooked Veg.
Fruit
Misc.
Milk

Date _____

Time   What I Ate

Meat
Bread
Cooked Veg.
Fruit
Misc.
Milk

Date _____

Time   What I Ate

Meat
Bread
Cooked Veg.
Fruit
Misc.
Milk

Figure 2-C
Food Diary for 1500 Calorie Diet

Date _____

Time   What I Ate

Meat
Bread
Cooked Veg.
Fruit
Misc.
Milk

Date _____

Time   What I Ate

Meat
Bread
Cooked Veg.
Fruit
Misc.
Milk

Date _____

Time   What I Ate

Meat
Bread
Cooked Veg.
Fruit
Misc.
Milk

Date _____

Time   What I Ate

Meat
Bread
Cooked Veg.
Fruit
Misc.
Milk

Figure 3
Hourly Success Chart

Hour	Monday	Tuesday	Wednesday	Thursday	Friday	Saturday	Sunday
6:00							
7:00							
8:00							
9:00							
10:00							
11:00							
12:00							
1:00							
2:00							
3:00							
4:00							
5:00							
6:00							
7:00							
8:00							
9:00							
10:00							
11:00							

THREE

Food Cues

D o YOU KNOW that often you eat not because you are depressed, bored, or lonely, but just because you saw the food? You wanted it and you ate it. It's as simple as that.

Anything that makes you want to eat is called a food cue. Imagine that you have just returned home from a late evening meeting. Everyone is in bed. You walk into the kitchen to shut off the light. You are not even thinking of eating. Suddenly you see a pan of brownies sitting on the counter, half-eaten, with the knife still in the pan. You will probably eat one, two, or many more. You are simply eating in response to a cue. You were not thinking of food. But you see the brownies and you eat them.

People with weight problems are especially sensitive to food cues. These cues do not affect thin people the same way. My husband can walk into the kitchen, see cookies on the counter, and think, "Oh, I guess we're having cookies for dessert tonight." He does not respond to a food cue in the same way that I might.

The best way to learn to control food cues is first of all to realize that they exist. Once you do this, you can begin to notice how you respond to them. If you fail to understand the way food cues operate, you will continue to eat a lot more than you intend, without knowing why.

Your goal should be to eliminate the food cues that cause you trouble. Of course you will not be able to eliminate every single one of them, but you can at least eliminate those in your immediate personal environment.

Your home should be a safe place for you. No matter how hard it is to diet when you are away from home, you should have the assurance that you can stick to your diet at home.

How to Make Your Home Safe

Step 1: Go through the house and collect food, bringing all of it to the kitchen, including the candy dish in the living room, the peanuts in the den, and the crackers by your bed. Let nothing escape your notice.

Step 2: Throw out the things you do not need or want. It is best to toss them down the garbage disposal if you have one. Get rid of those stale cookies that have been in the cupboard for six months and that half-eaten box of candy left over from Christmas. Throw out that old carton of ice cream in the freezer that has only three tablespoons left. Do it quickly and decisively. If you let yourself linger over it too long, you may end up falling for yet another food cue.

Step 3: Now clean up the kitchen. Make sure that the food is out of sight. Remember, food itself is the most powerful cue. Put into the cupboards everything that used to be on the counters. Get rid of the cookie jar. Even if it is empty, it still acts as a cue. Whenever you look at it, you will probably think, "cookie." Put it in the cupboard. If you really do not use it anymore, give it away, or just throw it away. Ideally, you should be able to walk into your kitchen without being hit by constant cues.

Step 4: Go the grocery store. Stock up on all the things that are going to help you stick to your diet—appealing fruits, fresh vegetables, diet pop, low-calorie salad dressings, items to make low-calorie treats, sugarless gum and mints, and so on. These will work as positive cues. If low-calorie foods are readily available and high-calorie foods are not, you will find it much easier to stick to your diet.

Consider this scenario. You decide that you are going to have a cup of tea and a nice, crisp apple as soon you get home from work. But when you open the refrigerator, you discover that the apples are all gone. However, you cast your eye on the leftover cheesecake from Saturday night. The outcome is predictable. If you really want to make a go at your diet, you should guard against such situations. It is your responsibility to make it easy for yourself to stay on your diet, not virtually impossible.

What about Treats for Family Members?

You may be fortunate enough to live in a household where everyone decides to go on a diet at the same time. That way no one will have to face the irresistible food cues that others might produce.

But it is more likely that you are doing this on your own. Perhaps you need to lose some weight, but your husband or your wife does not. What about treats for them? Let them have their treats. But make sure that these treats are not *your* favorites. Then see to it that they get put away in one particular cupboard, out of sight.

As a general rule, don't bake or ask others to bake for you. It is very easy to rationalize baking. "These are my children's favorite cookies." "My wife loves to cook for me." "My husband enjoys this pie. I want him to know how much I love him." Do not use food as a way of showing love. You cannot afford to. It simply gets you into too much trouble. There are lots of other ways to show love rather than by baking pies. Be creative. Look for ways to love people that are not food related. Give flowers. Write a kind note. Offer to fix something in need of repair. Make a gift. Do someone a special favor.

Instead of volunteering to bring the dessert to the wedding shower, bring the salad or the paper plates. Baking is a very strong food cue. Some women have been baking since they were children, and they have probably been reinforced for it on two counts. One, they are always thanked and praised for their wonderful treats. Two, they can eat some of the tasty ingredients while they are baking and they can share in the end product.

It is hard to give up all that positive reinforcement, but it is well worth it. In the end, it makes life so much easier for you.

Can I Ever Bake Again?

That is up to you. If you do, proceed with caution. When baking for a particular occasion, make just enough to insure that there won't be a lot of leftovers. It is the leftovers that can get you into trouble. If your wife is an avid baker, explain to her that it will help you if she bakes less while you are on your diet.

Perhaps friends invite you and your wife to dinner to celebrate your birthday. Everyone has a nice time. You have a piece of cake and feel fine about it. But you make the mistake of taking the leftover cake home. You eat some for lunch the next day, and then again for an afternoon snack, and then after dinner. The next day there is still one slice left, so you have it with your morning coffee. It would have been better to have left the cake with your well-meaning friends or to have given it to the neighbor, or simply to have thrown it out. It served its purpose—to help celebrate your birthday. It is of very little nutritional value, and it will not help you to have it around. It's not the one piece of dessert that causes trouble, but the leftovers.

Perhaps you have made fruitcakes for Christmas for the past fourteen years, and everyone in the family expects them again this year. Well, yes, it is true that you nibble a bit while you are making them. And yes, you do remember the year when you ate a whole one at one sitting just to sample it. You don't have to make fruitcakes any more. This is the year to break the tradition and come up with a new idea. You need to. It is probably just too risky to do it again. There are lots of other things that you can give for Christmas that will be just as appreciated.

The Office

The cupboards in your kitchen are clean and the food is out of sight. You have stocked up on your favorite fruits and vegetables. But what about the office? One of the secretaries keeps a jar of candy on her desk just for people to nibble on. Your boss brings in fresh donuts every Friday morning. Various companies send boxes of candy every so often as a gesture of goodwill. Is there anything you can do about it?

Everyone in my office is careful about their weight and physical fitness. Last Christmas a local pharmacist delivered a five-pound box of chocolates to the office on my day off. The staff decided among themselves to give it away to a group of bachelors, who were delighted to receive it. No one in the office would ever bring in high-calorie treats, except on rare occasions. Everyone there knows that treats are usually not appreciated.

Unfortunately, you probably do not work in such an ideal situation. It will take thought and diplomacy but you can do things to change your work environment. Start by surveying your situation. Brainstorm about what could be done. Perhaps all the food could be confined to an area that you could conscientiously avoid. You might talk to the secretary who keeps the candy on her desk and explain that you are trying to lose weight. Maybe she could keep the candy somewhere else. Be diplomatic. Don't insist on your way. If you handle it well, people will cooperate with you. Talk to your boss about the problem and ask whether he or she has any suggestions. Ask people not to offer you food. And then be persistent. Your co-workers may be very supportive for a week or two but then slowly revert to their old ways. Remind them that you are still on your diet and that you need all the help you can get.

More Cues

Be on the lookout for food cues. They are everywhere. Don't go to your favorite pizza restaurant anymore. Chances are it has become a cue for you to fill up on pizza and beer. If you find it impossible to simply order salad and coffee while you are there, it is probably best to avoid it for the time being. Try another restaurant where you can order salad and coffee with relatively little difficulty. You won't have the memories to cope with.

Avoid stopping at your favorite bakery for a cup of coffee. Instead, try the snack bar down the street that doesn't even sell baked goods. If you have to walk down the street the bakery is on, walk on the other side of the street. Don't cast a glance in the window as you pass by. You will only be asking for trouble.

Movie theaters can also present problems. For many people, going to the movies means food. For the past twenty years they have eaten popcorn everytime they have gone to the theater.

Has this been your habit? If so, you will find it difficult to say no to yourself when you are at a movie. You could stop attending movies entirely, or you could decide to go at a different time of the day than you are used to. If you do go, make sure that you have eaten a meal shortly before so that you aren't hungry. Get some coffee or a diet pop to drink. Chew gum. Bring a piece of fruit for a snack.

What about the nice little girl who comes to your door selling cookies? Pay for a box, if you want to, and ask her to give it to someone who cannot afford it. But do not make the mistake of bringing a box into the house, even if you don't intend to eat it. Many of my patients have eaten a whole box of cookies at one sitting just because a nice little girl brought it to their door. They weren't expecting it at that moment, and their defenses were down. These same people would never think of going to the grocery store and buying a box of cookies. They have learned how to deal with that situation, but they have not thought about how to deal with the little girl at the door until it is too late.

Do not hesitate to throw food away. Many of us have been raised with the notion that it is a sin to waste food. Of course it is wrong to be careless about food, but if you are overweight the best approach may be to get rid of high-calorie food. Very often, this food is of little nutritional value anyway. Just because you started eating that candy bar doesn't mean that you have to finish it. Throw it away. If you are eating something you know you should not be, get rid of it as fast as you can and walk away from it. You will walk away feeling victorious rather than defeated. If you eat something and there is only one bite left, throw that one bite away. Every time you do this, you will become more confident about your ability to resist high-calorie foods.

Learning how to recognize and control food cues is a very helpful tool. Doing it well takes wisdom and personal strength. It is not a sign of weakness to avoid the things that make you want to eat. On the contrary, it is a way of making wise decisions in your strong moments that will help you tremendously in your weak moments. And those weak moments are sure to come for all of us. The goal is to control your environment rather than letting it control you.

Week Three Assignment:

This week, in addition to keeping the food diary (see example at the end of chapter 2) every day and checking off your food exchanges as you use them, write down each day two examples of what you did to control food cues. You can write this at the bottom of your food diary for that day. Here are some examples:

—Some cookies were left on the counter. I put them in the cupboard as soon as I saw them.
—I refused to bring the leftover dessert home when it was offered.
—I talked with a friend in the living room rather than in the kitchen, where I am more likely to eat.
—I placed the potato chips on the opposite side of the table from me.
—I removed the peanut butter from the top shelf of the refrigerator to the cupboard, so I will not see it when I open the refrigerator for the water pitcher.
—I threw out the remaining pudding. I was home alone and knew I would eat it otherwise.

—I avoided the hors d'oeuvres at the party.

—I threw away the kids' leftover desserts immediately, rather than eating them.

FOUR

Sit Down and Slow Down

W E ARE CUED to eat by a variety of things—the brownies left out on the kitchen counter, tempting magazine ads, persuasive TV commercials, and many other things. A subtle but powerful cue is that of place. If you frequently eat in the same place, that place itself becomes a cue.

Consider, for example, a traveling salesman who keeps food in his car and frequently eats while driving. Before long, the mere act of getting into the car will be a cue or stimulus that will make him want to eat, regardless of whether there is any food in the car.

Many people eat standing up in the kitchen, usually while cooking or cleaning up. For these people, simply standing in the kitchen can become a strong cue to eat. I remember one patient whose favorite place to eat was back in one corner of her kitchen, where she couldn't be seen from the street. This was her secret eating place. After she began dieting, she found that this "place" was a very strong cue for her. Every time she saw it, she wanted to eat.

Many students sit down to their desks to study, well-stocked with snacks and drinks. Studying then becomes a cue to eating. It can become impossible for them to sit at their desk without thinking of food.

Watching TV can also be a very potent cue. For years you may have spent several evenings each week watching TV and eating an endless variety of snacks. Just sitting down to watch TV has become a cue.

The list is endless. Any place where you frequently eat can in itself become a cue—your bed, the office desk, the lounge at work, your sewing room, the bowling alley, the grocery store.

Your Designated Eating Place

Choose a place where you will eat all of your meals and snacks. We will call this your designated eating place. It should be an appropriate eating place, like the dining room table, the kitchen table, or both. It is all right to drink liquids at other places, but whenever you eat, you should sit at your designated place.

You should also choose a designated eating place at work. Don't choose your office desk, if at all possible. Instead, choose the cafeteria, lounge, or some other place that you can use only for eating.

Other places can also serve temporarily as your designated eating place, for instance, a restaurant, a picnic, and so on. You may decide to have guests over for a buffet dinner in the living room. At that time, the living room would be the appropriate eating place. But under normal circumstances, it would be out of bounds.

Your car is not an appropriate eating place, nor is the movie theater. If you are cooking dinner and want to nibble on something, fix a small plate and sit down at your eating place. At this point, it is better to eat a cookie at your eating place than an apple standing up in the kitchen.

This technique can make your eating habits less impulsive. If you really want something, you will have to sit down and eat it. If you are just impulsively grabbing it, you will think twice before eating it.

If you do this consistently for anywhere from one to three months, your old "eating places" will lose their power as food cues. You will be able to watch television for hours without thinking about eating. The car will no longer make you want a snack. The dining room and kitchen table will be food cues, but that is appropriate.

You will want to continue this technique for the rest of your life. You may not always need to be quite so rigid about it, but if you start becoming too lenient with yourself, you will want to go back to your original program for a while.

Slow Down

Are you always the first one finished with dinner? Are you on seconds when everyone else has just finished their first serving? Can you easily eat an egg salad sandwich in less than one minute and a full dinner in less than fifteen minutes? If you are overweight, you probably eat twice as fast as your thin counterpart. This means that you may eat twice as much. If you want to lose weight and keep it off, you will need to change the rate at which you eat.

Most of us have developed a very efficient way of eating. We begin by taking a bite; while chewing it, we fill our fork, moving it close to our mouth. As soon as that first bite starts to go down, we insert the second. This process continues quite rapidly until all the food is gone. We need to slow down.

Several years ago I had dinner with a couple who are good friends of mine. The husband is extremely thin. That particular night we ate tuna sandwiches. I happened to notice how long it was taking people to eat. The husband took no less than forty-five minutes to eat one tuna sandwich! I was amazed. He would take a bite, put the sandwich back down on his plate, wipe his mouth with his napkin, and then talk for five minutes before returning to his sandwich. At times he even seemed to forget that it was there at all. His eating pattern was not deliberate, but it was a major reason why he was so thin.

This is an exaggerated pattern and not one that you need to strive for. I want to offer you a few techniques to help you slow down, make the food last longer, and enable you to enjoy it more.

Put Your Fork Down

The best way to begin eating slowly is to put your fork down between bites. Don't refill it until you have chewed and swallowed the food in your mouth. Then, and only then, pick up your fork, put some food on it, and take the next bite. Repeat this process until you have eaten all the food on your plate.

The way to develop this habit is to grade yourself. If you put your food down after every single bite, give yourself an "A" in a new column on your food diary. We will call this your "eating slowly" column. If you put your fork down only between every other bite, then you give yourself a "B." If you completely forgot to put your fork or spoon down, give yourself an "F." If you are eating a sandwich, an apple, or some type of finger food, then you should put that down between each bite.

Try sipping water or some low-calorie drink between bites. Keep a pitcher of water on the table so that you can easily refill your glass. If you have to get up and go to the kitchen, you are less likely to sip between bites.

It helps to make mealtimes a quiet, relaxed, and peaceful experience. Put on some soft music. Use candles or soft lighting. Take care to set the table nicely. Make meal times, especially dinner time, a pleasant, enjoyable time. If you rush in from a busy day, hurry through dinner, and go off to a class or meeting, you are going to find it very difficult to eat slowly. Perhaps you have noticed that when you go out for an evening with friends, everyone tends to eat more slowly, to relax and enjoy the food. It is much easier to eat slowly in a relaxed and pleasant atmosphere.

Of course you cannot spend the whole evening every evening eating dinner, but you can do some things which will make the meal time peaceful and relaxing. Try to have dinner ready ahead of time so that you are not rushing around at the last minute. If you are, you will sit down to dinner tense and tired.

It helps to drink something a few minutes before dinner. Try a glass of tomato juice or vegetable juice or a cup of boullion or tea. It will take the edge off your hunger and help you to relax before actually eating your meal.

Give yourself some kind of cue to remind yourself to eat slowly. One simple way to do this is to make a little "cue" card to put at your place at the table, saying "Slow Down." For a more subtle approach, lay your watch on the table by your plate and let it remind you to slow down. Or put your knife across your plate in such a way that it will act as a signal for you to eat more slowly. You will need a cue like this. It is all too easy to forget and to slip into the old habits.

Your main meal of the day should last at least twenty minutes. If you eat slowly and drink liquids between bites, it will last at least that long and probably longer. A helpful technique involves taking a two-minute break at some point during the meal. I usually do this after I have eaten most, though not all, of my dinner. Put your fork down, sit back, and time yourself. Wait two full minutes. Some people actually find it necessary to get up and walk around when they first begin doing this. That's okay. Sit on your hands if you have to. Go put water on for coffee. Do whatever helps, but stop eating for two full minutes. When the time is up, go back to the food. Sometimes people find this technique so helpful that they use it twice in one meal. Many thin people do this naturally.

Keep track of this in your "eating slowly" column. If you took your two-minute break at your main meal, indicate it by a "2." If you forgot or failed to do it for some reason, put a "-2" in the column. Do this for at least one week. If you like it, and it seems helpful to you, then continue it.

Other Helps

Never use soup spoons. Use a teaspoon to eat your soup or cereal. It will help you slow down. For the same reason, use a salad fork instead of a regular fork.

Certain foods and drinks can help slow you down and make the meal last longer. Give yourself plenty of food. Just be sure to choose the right things. If your dinner consists of a four-ounce piece of meat loaf, a small baked potato and a small apple, you will use up all your exchanges without being very satisfied. If, instead, dinner consists of a cup of boullion, a large lettuce salad with low-calorie dressing, a large serving of green beans, four ounces of meat loaf, a small baked potato, iced tea, a small apple, and a cup of coffee, you will probably be quite satisfied and take much longer to eat. Always include vegetables and liquids with your meals. For lunch, I usually recommend some type of raw vegetable, a salad, or carrot and celery sticks, or the equivalent. At dinner, always plan at least one cooked vegetable and possibly two, along with a salad.

Choose foods that you can eat in substantial portions. For instance, plan on a cup of strawberries rather than two tablespoons of raisins. They are both equal to one fruit exchange, but the strawberries are going to be a lot more filling.

The Chocolate Milk Shake Experiment

Jean Mayer, a Harvard nutritionist, developed an experiment to try to determine what it is that makes us say we are "full." Is it the amount of calories we have eaten or the volume we have taken in?

He began by asking his subjects to exercise. When they had finished, he gave them a chocolate milk shake to drink. The milk shake was in an opaque container so that they could not tell how much they were drinking. He was able to increase the calorie content by ten times before they could tell a difference in the taste. He found that people felt full or satiated based on how much they had had to drink, not on how many calories they take in. Thus, we sense fullness by volume, not by how many calories we take in.

You can take advantage of this knowledge by making sure that you always you have plenty of low-calorie food to eat. To lose weight, you don't have to scrimp on the quantity you eat. You can eat a very satisfying amount of food if you select wisely from your diet.

Slowing the rate of your eating can significantly affect the amount you eat. It is worth training yourself and your family to slow down. Keep track in your food diary of how fast you eat and of how faithfully you take your two-minute break. These are techniques that you should continue using throughout the diet. Begin to use reasonable quantities of low-calorie foods to supplement your meals and snacks. There is no reason why you need to walk away from the table hungry or unsatisfied. Make your meals sufficient, pleasant, and satisfying. It may take a little more time to do this, but it's well worth it.

Week Four Assignment:

1. Use figure 4 to keep track of your eating places this week. Every time you sit down to eat at one of your designated eating places, check the appropriate box. If you eat anywhere else, check that box. Your goal should be to draw a straight line all the way across under your designated eating place.
2. Continue keeping your food diary throughout the diet. Check off your exchanges this week.
3. Add a column to your food diary labeled "eating slowly." Each time you eat, rate how slowly you ate and enter your grade in the column. Indicate whether you took a two-minute break by a "2" or a "-2." Use low-calorie foods and liquids in sufficient quantity at meals to help yourself feel full.

Figure 4

Eating Place Record

(Numbers under the days of the week refer to consecutive eating episodes)

Place	Monday 1 2 3 4 5 6	Tuesday 1 2 3 4 5 6	Wednesday 1 2 3 4 5 6	Thursday 1 2 3 4 5 6	Friday 1 2 3 4 5 6	Saturday 1 2 3 4 5 6	Sunday 1 2 3 4 5 6
Car							
Office desk							
Den—TV room							
Living room							
Designated eating place							
Bedroom							
Kitchen (not at table)							
Other							

FIVE

Impulses and How They Work

A FEW YEARS AGO I was working in an office near a small ice cream and candy shop. I would frequently run nextdoor for a treat. One day my boss asked me if I would go over to the shop and get him some ice cream sometime that week. "Sometime that week!" I could not imagine it. When I wanted ice cream, I wanted it right then, not a week later.

That was the beginning of a long series of lessons in which I learned to recognize my impulses and to make definite rational decisions about whether to give in to them.

Our impulses are similar to demanding children. The more we reward or reinforce them, the more demands they make. The less we reinforce them, the more trained and disciplined they will become.

Consider what happens when a mother is raising a child. Let's say that Mom is cooking dinner. Johnny comes in and asks politely for a cookie. Mom says, "No, you can't have a cookie until after dinner." Johnny is not put off by this and stands by her, whining and pulling at her skirt, begging for a cookie. Finally, Mom gives in. She has just reinforced his whining behavior. That was the farthest thing from her intention. She was simply trying to keep him quiet and get him out of the kitchen. But by giving in, she is training Johnny that asking politely for a cookie gets no results. It is more effective to whine and to demand what he wants.

Our impulses are much the same. If we always say yes to our urge for a cookie, then we are training ourselves to give in whenever we feel like eating. Even though many of our impulses may be out of line, it's not too late to get them into shape. If you want to train your eating impulses, the first thing to do is to delay gratifying them. You want to teach them that they will not always get what they want immediately. When an urge to eat hits, it is usually very strong and demanding. If you can just make it wait a few minutes, its strength will often diminish, and you will be able to control it more effectively.

Suppose that you are at the office, hard at work on a project. You get up for a cup of coffee, not even thinking about food. Right next to the coffee pot is an open box of donuts. As soon as you see them, you want one. But you decide to make yourself wait for fifteen minutes. Remind yourself that you can live without a donut for fifteen minutes. Go sit down at your desk and get back to work. You will find that after fifteen minutes, you will no longer feel such a strong urge to eat. It will be much easier for you to decide not to eat the donuts at all. But if you absolutely must have a donut, go ahead and get one. At least you did not reinforce the impulse immediately. You made it wait a few minutes. And that is the first step to making it wait a day, a week, and sometimes to saying no entirely.

Try practicing this technique even with the things you can have, like a cup of coffee or a stick of gum. It's 3:00 and you want a cup of coffee. Say to yourself, "Okay, I can have some coffee, but I am going to wait until 3:30 for it." Your goal is to reach the point at which all your impulses are under your control. You should be able to tell them exactly what they are to have and when.

This delaying technique can be especially effective at night. You may be on your way to bed, when suddenly you get the idea that you would like a cup of hot chocolate. Tell yourself to go to bed. Say to yourself that you can have it in the morning if you still want it. Then go on to bed. Chances are that by the next morning you will have forgotten your desire. Even if you do remember it, a cup of hot chocolate probably will not sound all that appealing to you.

When the impulse comes, it will usually make a false promise or lie to you. "Just one cookie. All I want is one cookie and then I will be satisfied." But you know what happens. You give in and have one cookie. Very soon it is back again saying, "Just one more cookie. That's all I want." At some point you are going to have to say, "No, that's it. Now, leave me alone." It is just as easy to say no at the beginning as it is after several cookies.

When you say no in the beginning, you are not just avoiding fifty or one hundred calories. You are refusing to reinforce the impulse. In doing so you are beginning to train and discipline it. If you give in, it will be that much harder to resist it the next time.

Week Five Assignment:

Use the food impulse chart in figure 5 to keep track of all your food impulses this week. Record the number of times the impulse to eat hits you, the number of times you successfully resisted it, and the number of times you gave in. You will observe that in the first week you may experience many food impulses. As you say no to them, refusing to give in to them, you will notice that they occur less and less.

You must also use the other techniques you have learned, especially cue elimination. As long as a cookie is sitting in front of you, you are going to continue to want it. But if you remove it or remove yourself from the situation, the impulse will leave you alone.

Figure 5
Training Food Impulses

Day	Number of Impulses to Eat	Said No	Said Yes
Monday			
Tuesday			
Wednesday			
Thursday			
Friday			
Saturday			
Sunday			

SIX

Don't Overcompensate

WHENEVER WE FEEL DEPRIVED, we tend to overeat. And we tend to feel most deprived whenever we skip a meal.

Let's say that you are doing well on your diet. You are busy at work and lunchtime rolls around. You say to yourself, "I think I'll skip lunch today. I'm not even hungry, and that way I'll lose weight even faster." It sounds like a good idea. But 4:30 arrives and you are starving. As soon as you get home, you decide that you deserve a snack. After all, you did skip lunch. You end up eating too much, consuming more calories than you would have if you had eaten a normal lunch at noon.

One of the cardinal rules of successful dieting is to avoid missing meals. Whatever you do, *don't skip meals*. Think of your meals as you would think of medicine. If you were taking medicine for high blood pressure, you would not skip the noon dose just because you did not feel like taking it. By the same token, do not eat or refrain from eating just because you feel like it. Skipping meals usually leads to overeating.

It is easy to feel deprived when everyone else is eating something appetizing and you are not. Perhaps there was cake for last night's dessert, and you turned it down. Later that night you snuck down to the kitchen and ate not just one piece of cake but several.

The best way to deal with such situations is to plan ahead. If you know that everyone else is going to have dessert, then plan a treat for yourself. You may only decide to have a cup of coffee.

But it is your decision. You thought about it in advance and that is what counts. Tell yourself that you could have dessert if you wanted it. You could eat ten pieces of cake if you liked. But you don't want to. You want to be thin. You don't want to be at the mercy of that little impulse that demands whatever it sees. Who is the boss? You or your impulses? You, of course. When that little impulse starts giving you a hard time, talk to it just like you would to a child. Just because it demands something does not mean that it is going to get it. *You* are the one running the show, not the impulse. It's important to tell yourself that you could have the food if you wanted, but that you are choosing not to have it because you want to be thin. You are not deprived. You are simply making a better choice.

I'm Tired—I Need Something to Eat

Fatigue is a common cause of overeating. Have you ever been up at 11:00 P.M. and thought, "I'm so tired. If I could just eat something, I could keep going"? The wise thing would be to go to bed. You need regular, adequate amounts of sleep. If you refuse to get it, you will have a very difficult time following this or any diet. Don't resist sleep. Don't think of it as an imposition on your time and your day. Sleep is a blessing from the Lord, a time to be refreshed, not just physically, but spiritually. After a good night's sleep, you will often wake up with a fresh perspective. Difficulties that seemed utterly overwhelming the night before will shrink to manageable proportions.

Not only is it important to get enough sleep, but it is essential to get regular sleep. You are not doing yourself a favor by going to bed at 8:00 P.M. one night and midnight the next, even if you are getting eight hours of sleep both nights. When you do this, you are actually throwing your body into jet lag. You may become irritable, disoriented, fatigued, headachy, dizzy, and so on. It is not necessary to fly from Chicago to Rome to suffer jet lag; you can bring it on yourself simply by maintaining an erratic sleep schedule.

It is important, even essential, to establish a regular schedule for sleep and meals. You probably have some idea about what works best for you. But you may need to experiment before you find the right routine. Once you find it, don't vary it unless you must. The most important times of your day are when you get up in the morning, when you eat your meals, and when you go to bed. Feel free to vary your bedtime or rising time by an hour if you need to but never more than that, unless it is absolutely unavoidable. Do not base your meals and your sleep time around your busy schedule; instead, base your busy schedule around your meals and sleep time. Consider the sample schedule at the end of this chapter. Your schedule should serve you and your diet, not the reverse.

Sleep can also serve as a good escape from the temptation to eat. If it is 10:00 P.M. and you are starting to think about the crackers in the kitchen, just go to bed. Who can eat while they are sleeping? If naps help you, then take them. If it is 2:00 Saturday afternoon and you are tired and want to eat something to keep yourself going, consider taking a nap instead.

The Bored Eater

No one is home. You have nothing particular to do. Bored, you wander into the kitchen and look for something interesting to eat. Does this sound familiar? Don't let it happen again. Avoid boredom at all costs. It is death to your diet.

Have you ever heard someone say, "I got so busy I forgot to eat"? They are not lying. That actually does happen to many people. You may even be able to remember a few times when it has happened to you.

I am not suggesting that you should forget to eat, but only pointing out that you will be less likely to think of food if you are busy and active. Busying yourself with different activities can help you delay reinforcing a food impulse. Sometimes you will become so occupied with various activities that you will experience less frequent impulses.

Do you have a lot of time on your hands? Do you find yourself easily bored? If so, you will need to look for ways to keep yourself busy, to fill up your schedule. Life is too short to waste time eating for lack of better things to do. If you are not currently working and have a lot of time on your hands, you may want to consider getting a full- or part-time job. You might be able to find some type of work that you could do at home.

Perhaps you have no trouble keeping busy during the day but become bored at night, spending countless hours watching TV and snacking. You could take an evening class or join a civic or church group. There are innumerable ways that you could volunteer to serve people in real need. It is important that you stay active and busy. Your life will be more satisfying to you, and you will be looking to food less to fill up the time.

Develop some of your hobbies and interests. Some pleasant, enjoyable activities should form part of your week. You needn't become engrossed in your hobby at the expense of family life or your relationship with the Lord, but you should do some things simply for fun and relaxation.

Some of the busiest people I know (and the thinnest) are the ones who take time for their hobbies. One friend of mine, the father of six children, is active in Christian service and holds a very responsible job. Even with all these commitments, he takes time out for his hobbies. If he has a few free hours, he will grab his gun and his dogs and go hunting. He doesn't spend every weekend at it, but he fits it in when he can.

Another friend of mine has a dog that he loves. When he gets home from work, he takes the dog for a walk or spends time brushing it. It doesn't take hours, only a few minutes here and there.

Allow yourself to find pleasure and relaxation in things other than food. Food should never be your only source of pleasure. You should relate to it primarily as a source of nutrition. The trouble comes when you expect too much from it. Of course food will always be pleasurable, but it should not be one of the main sources of pleasure in your life.

Brouse through the library or a bookstore. Look for books on areas that interest you. "How to" books can be a good place to start. Take a class that interests you: knitting, gardening, computers, calligraphy, swimming, carpentry, oil painting, history, or something else. But, whatever you do, don't take a cooking class. It will usually just contribute to the problem rather than help.

Activities can help you deal with immediate food impulses. Make a list of possible activities. Include activities you can do in five minutes, activities that take longer, and some activities that take a whole afternoon or evening. List pleasant, relaxing activities, such as writing a letter, calling a friend, going fishing, going shopping. Also include chores and tasks that need to be done: mow the lawn, paint the garage, clean the basement, do the laundry, and so on. Include in this list some tasks that aren't part of your weekly routine.

Keep the list handy, taping it to the refrigerator, or leaving it on a desk or dresser. Put it in an obvious place where you will see it frequently. Having done this, you can use the list in two ways.

First of all, you can use it whenever a food impulse hits. For example, you have finished dinner and have been sitting on the sofa reading the paper for the last forty-five minutes. You get up, slightly bored, wander into the kitchen, and look for something to eat. It is at just such a time that you should look at your activity list and tell yourself that you are going to go do at least one of the things on the list before you eat anything. Once you become involved in the activity, you will probably forget about eating. You were not really hungry in the first place, only bored.

A second way to make use of your activity list is to refer to it *before* the food impulse hits. Suppose that it is Saturday afternoon. You had to postpone your golf game because of heavy rains. Instead of wandering around the house, bored, look at your list and choose a substitute activity. Get involved in it before you have a chance to think about food. Choose an activity that appeals to you, one that you will enjoy. If you choose something that you don't really want to do, like cleaning out the garage, you are more likely to turn to food to help you procrastinate. Choose something that sounds interesting, fun, or challenging.

Your Schedule and How to Make It Work

Your daily schedule and your diet may seem totally unrelated. But a well-functioning schedule can make a big difference to the success and ease with which you diet. Using the sample schedule in figure 6, write in the times when you will get up in the morning, eat breakfast, lunch, and dinner, and go to bed at night. You should base the rest of your day around those times. Don't base those times around the rest of your day. If you are going to be out shopping on Saturday, one of the first things you should plan is when and where you will stop for lunch. Don't wait until three o'clock to say to yourself, "I'm starving. Where can I get something to eat?" Under such circumstances you will probably choose the wrong kind of place and almost certainly go off your diet.

Once you have written in your mealtimes and your bedtime, fill in the rest of your schedule with the other things that you need to do this week. If you are working forty hours a week, a good deal of time is already scheduled for you, but plan what you want to do in the evenings and on the weekends. Set aside at least one evening a week for personal time. Spend it any way you like. Read your favorite book. Write a letter. Be sure to use that one evening to take care of your personal needs, or just to relax. If an evening does not work for you, then take a morning or a few hours in the afternoon. It is usually best to plan on a night during the week rather than on the weekend, since weekends can be busy and difficult to predict. Having that kind of time built into your week can serve as a way to refresh you. It can make you less likely to turn to food for refreshment. But it will not happen automatically. You will have to plan it.

On your schedule, plan what you will be doing each night of the week. Do not let an evening go by in which you did not know what you were going to do beforehand. If you fail to plan, you will be setting yourself up for boredom. Chances are that you will end up in the kitchen.

The activities that you choose should have nothing to do with food. Cooking may have been one of your hobbies in the past.

Put that behind you. You will need to develop other hobbies—refinishing furniture, golfing, sewing, or gardening. Look for things that interest you but that have nothing at all to do with food.

Week Six Assignment:

1. Record the actual time you go to bed and the time you get up every day for one week. Calculate the total number of hours you sleep each night. Are you getting enough sleep to make you feel your best? Are your bed times regular?
2. Draw up an activity list and post it in a convenient place.
3. Fill out your schedule for the next week. (See the sample in figure 6.)
4. Each day, write an example about how choosing an activity helped you deal with a food impulse. Write it at the bottom of your food diary. For example, "I was bored and wanted to eat but decided to re-pot some plants instead" or "I was frustrated at the office and wanted a candy bar, but decided to go for a brief walk instead."

My Activity List

1. Write Mom
2. Clean fish tank
3. Play the piano
4. Go to the library
5. Do yard work
6. Work on budget
7. Play racquetball
8. Work in darkroom
9. Listen to music
10. Go for a bike ride with the kids

Figure 6
My Schedule for the Week of _____

Monday		Tuesday		Wednesday		Thursday		Friday		Saturday		Sunday	
Time	Activity	Time	Activity	Time	Activity	Time	Activity	Time	Activity	Time	Activity	Time	Activity
	Get Up		Get Up		Get Up		Get Up		Get Up		Get Up		Get Up
	Breakfast		Breakfast		Breakfast		Breakfast		Breakfast		Breakfast		Breakfast
	Lunch		Lunch		Lunch		Lunch		Lunch		Lunch		Lunch
	Dinner		Dinner		Dinner		Dinner		Dinner		Dinner		Dinner
	Bedtime		Bedtime		Bedtime		Bedtime		Bedtime		Bedtime		Bedtime

SEVEN

Advertising Psychology and Why It Makes Us Fat

THE PRODUCTION AND MARKETING of food is big business. Make no mistake about it. The goal of food advertisers is to sell you their products, regardless of whether you want them. Of course their first goal is to convince you that you do want or need whatever they are selling. Convincing consumers to buy is the purpose of all advertising. And the food industry is no exception. In fact, food and related corporations buy a tremendous volume of ad space on television and radio programs and in newspapers and magazines. In 1981, food corporations were the number one advertisers in terms of total dollars spent.[2]

You may be determined to lose weight, rid your home of food cues, and control your impulses. Overall, your diet may be going quite well, until you unwittingly fall into the hands of the food advertising industry. Under their influence and with the help of your impulses, you bring home a beautiful coffee cake that you got for half-price at the grocery store. You go to a restaurant and order a large breakfast with all the trimmings, instead of the toast you had planned on. You find yourself in the kitchen making a pizza after having watched the Saturday night movie. Are these lapses simply your own doing? Probably not.

People who specialize in advertising psychology make it their business to know what makes you buy food. And of course they use their discoveries to sell their products. Their expertise is great for profits but hard on your diet and your self-esteem. You need to make it your business to know their ploys, to alert yourself to them, and to learn a good defense.

Grocery Stores

Whenever you walk into a grocery store, you should have your guard up. Of course the food itself acts as a very powerful cue. But food manufacturers and grocery stores have additional techniques to convince you to buy their products.

It is of utmost importance to the manufacturer that his product is packaged in a way that captures your attention and persuades you to add the product to your shopping cart. This emphasis on attention-getting is hardly surprising since so many thousands of products compete for your dollars.

You may think that a grocery store is simply a large warehouse in which food is stored until purchased by the consumer. But, in fact, grocery stores are sophisticated enterprises, where food is carefully displayed for the consumer. True, the physical layout of the store is designed for convenience, but even more than that, it is designed to call maximum attention to attractive, high-profit items, often high-calorie items. The cardinal rule for the layout of any grocery story is to expose as much of the product as possible, because the rate of exposure is directly related to the rate of sales.[3] Clearly, the store owner knows how powerful food cues can be.

The products themselves are the salesmen. Simply let the customer see enough of it, make the product attractive, and it will sell itself. Therefore, the store planner must strive for maximum exposure by subtly guiding the shopper through each department in the store. Most stores locate the high profit departments around the periphery of the store, the area of the greatest traffic flow, thus creating more exposure for those high-profit items.

Did you ever wonder why milk is placed in the far, rear corner of the store, rather inconvienient if that is all you need? The reason is clear. Milk has very high drawing power. *Drawing* power is a term grocers use to indicate that a particular item is purchased by a very high percentage of their customers.[4] By placing it in the back of the store, the grocer insures that you will have to walk all the way through the store to get a quart of milk. He hopes you will be attracted to something you see on the shelves and end up purchasing a few more items that you intended.

The grocer is careful to place the high-profit impulse products near the products with drawing power. You reach to get something you need, and right next to it is something you do not need. But it looks so good. If your defenses are down, you may fall for the bait.

Over half the purchases that the average shopper makes are made on impulse. Does that surprise you? This is why high-impulse items show up in the most prominent places.

The amount of space allocated for various grocery products is determined both by the need to meet consumer demand and the desire to influence consumer demand. Studies indicate that there is a direct relationship between how many times a product is exposed on the front edge of the shelf and the sales of that item.[5]

Items that are stocked closest to eye level have a sales advantage over products located at waist or floor level. In one study, the sale of a certain brand of raisins increased by 67 percent when moved from floor to eye level.[6]

You may have noticed that most modern grocery stores have long, continuous aisles. Grocers know that having continuous shelving is more effective for sales than having cross-over aisles. Longer aisles mean more exposure.

Often, grocery stores will use gimmicks such as giving away small pieces of cheese or sausage on toothpicks. Some stores now have a small lunch counter where you can sit, relax, and have a bite to eat. The longer the store can keep you "in house," the greater the likelihood that you will spend more money.

The produce section contains a minimum of advertising gimmicks. After this section your cart is carefully guided into the baked goods area. Usually tables or shelves are set up in such a way that it is difficult to hurry through. You cannot simply pick up your loaf of bread without also noticing that there is a special this week on apple pie, two for the price of one. Of course it had not occurred to you to buy even one apple pie, much less two. But can you afford to pass up this special? The children love pie. You slip two into your basket and move on.

In the next aisle you expect to find a box of saltines. They are on the bottom shelf, and your eyes wander until they rest on an attractively packaged box of snack crackers, placed at eye level. They look so much more inviting and pleasant than the plain white and red saltine box, so into the cart they go. This process continues aisle after aisle, until you arrive at the checkout counter. But you are number five in line and everyone ahead of you seems to be buying enough groceries for an army. You brace yourself for a twenty-minute wait. But immediately you fall victim to the table of "sale" items set up next to the line. Valentine candy is on sale at 40% off. What a bargain! It, too, goes into the cart. As you approach the cashier, you notice a display of candy bars. You realize that you are hungry. After all, you have been working hard and deserve a treat. So you pick up a candy bar that looks especially good. You have to judge from the wrapper, of course, since you cannot see what is inside. You decide to eat it and pay the clerk for the empty package. Finally, your turn comes. She checks you out, loads the cart, and you leave the store behind for another week.

Food manufacturers and grocers are not villains, deliberately trying to make you fat. They are simply trying to generate a nice profit. They are not malicious or underhanded, but merely smart businessmen who know what works. But the truth is that profit for them can mean fat for you.

Strategy for Grocery Shopping

Armed with this knowledge, how should you approach grocery shopping? Here are a few tips.

1. Approach grocery shopping as work, not fun. Consider it part of your job. Plan something else for fun. Try to shop as

quickly as possible. The longer you are in the store, the greater the likelihood that you will succumb to food cues or advertising gimmicks.

2. Make a shopping list. Know exactly what you are going to buy. It will help if you plan your menus a week or two at a time. Once you have chosen your menus, make as accurate a grocery list as possible and shop directly from it. I use what I call a master marketing list (explained in detail in chapter 10). You can draw up a similar list for yourself. Before going grocery shopping, simply check off what you need and write in any extras. Such a list will prevent you from forgetting things and help you avoid an extra trip to the grocery store.

3. Never shop on an empty stomach. Go grocery shopping right after a meal so that you will not be hungry. It's hard enough to face the grocery store on a full stomach. Never go when you are famished. If you do, you will be putting yourself to the test unnecessarily, and you might fail.

4. Avoid eye contact with certain foods. Don't even look at the bakery section. All it takes is a split-second glance to plant the desire in your mind. Look at the floor or at the ceiling, but refuse to look at what is on the shelves. Avoid certain aisles if you can. Avoid the candy aisle and the deli if possible.

5. Refrain from buying anything that might cause you trouble. If donuts are too much of a temptation, don't buy them. Buy English muffins instead, or something you handle better.

The chocolate-cream cookies are on sale. You glanced up and just happened to notice them. Maybe the children would like some. Ask yourself who they are really for. Be honest. Perhaps the children do not even like chocolate-cream cookies all that much. If you have to buy them a treat, buy something you don't care for, or give them some money and let them buy a treat at school. But never deliberately buy something that might prove a temptation for you.

6. Chew gum while you are in the store if that helps.

7. Go shopping with a friend if that helps.

8. Go to the grocery store as infrequently as possible. The

more you go, the more temptation you will face.

9. Try switching to a new store. If you have frequently purchased high-calorie food at a certain store, the store itself may have become a strong food cue. Try a new store, where you can start out fresh.

Promises, Promises

A convincing case could be made that food advertising is a major contributing factor to the prevalence of weight problems in our country. After all, a fixed number of people can consume only so much food. Since the market is not constantly expanding, the manufacturer must advertise heavily if he wants to keep his product in the forefront of the customer's mind. Unfortunately, you and I are casualties in the ensuing war between the advertisers.

Positioning is a term used by advertisers to describe the way a particular product or service is placed, or "positioned," in the customer's mind. For instance, a certain brand of soup may be positioned in such a way that it always conjures up warm lunches on cold winter days, loving mothers, happy children, and so on. Positioning is achieved by advertising the product in a particular way over a period of time, usually using a variety of media and methods: TV spots, magazine ads, store displays, coupons, free samples. If the campaign was successful, the product is positioned in our minds in exactly the way the advertisers intended.

Effective advertising always carries a promise. Of course, no one is going to promise you that you will get fat if you eat their products. Instead, the advertisers promise things like fun, attractiveness, homeyness, a happy family. After all, you deserve it, don't you? Whatever promise will sell the product is the one that is promoted.

The aim of any effective ad is to grab your attention and keep it. How else will you get the message unless you see the same advertisement again and again? Repetition means retention. The goal is to fix the product firmly in your mind so that when you see it you will choose it over the competition.

It can help to be aware of some of the advertising techniques in common use. Here are some of them:

—Identification with characters. The ad portrays someone you can relate to, the housewife, the sports enthusiast, the businessman.

—Demonstration. The ad shows what the product does, how to use it, and how effective it is.

—Humor. The ad makes you laugh. The implication is that if you buy this food, you will have fun.

—Catchy slogans. These usually employ rhyme or rhythm. They help the consumer remember the product.

Ads range from clever to obnoxious. Some make use of sexual innuendo and others feature celebrities—anything to make us remember the product at the crucial moment: when we come face to face with it at the supermarket.

Television and magazine ads often make food look bigger, better, and more delicious than the real thing. Consumer incentives can help sell products that have trouble selling on their own merits or ones that face stiff competition. All of us are familiar with the following gimmicks: a premium (a free set of measuring spoons if you buy this cake mix); a bargain; a free sample (either in the mail or at the store); a chance to win something.

Defending Yourself

Make it your business to know what the advertisers are up to. If you realize that you are considering buying Brand X for no other reason than the commercial you saw last night, that knowledge will help you walk right past it.

Second, look at television commercials objectively. Try to stay a bit aloof from them rather than letting them take you in. Turn the sound down during advertisements. Limit your TV watching. Television and radio commercials can act as exceptionally strong food cues. Whatever you do, resist eating in response to them.

Third, never dwell on food ads in magazines and newspapers. The longer you look at the ad, the more it will work on you. Don't bother reading the recipe connected with the pudding ad. It is probably not a recipe you should be using anyway.

Fourth, don't save coupons for food you know you should not be buying. Even if a coupon enables you to buy something for half price, don't buy it unless you would normally use it.

Fifth, never be enticed just because of a sale—even if something is being given away free. You don't want anything that will get your diet off track.

Lastly, don't fall for all the promises. Food cannot make you happy, and you know it. Remember that food manufacturing and advertising is a multi-billion dollar business. It is a lot to fight against. But you can fight and you can win.

Week Seven Assignment:

1. Make a shopping list before you go to the store
2. Plan to go grocery shopping after a meal.
3. Go to the grocery store only once a week.
4. Continue your simple food diary and check off your food exchanges as you use them.

EIGHT

Exercise Is Essential

JEAN MAYER, THE NUTRITIONIST, noticed that his laboratory mice never seemed to get fat. They had an ever-present supply of food, but they always seemed to eat just the right amount to maintain their weights. He decided to do some experiments with them to see if they would lose weight if he made them exercise more. They didn't. They simply ate a little more food and maintained the same weight. He further increased the amount of exercise, but the mice simply ate more and kept their weight stable. So he began to decrease their exercise. As he did so, they decreased their food intake. He decreased the amount of exercise even further. They continued to eat less, until finally they reached a point of minimal exercise and began to overeat and gain weight. It seemed that the mice had some kind of innate balance between energy intake and energy output. As soon as they began exercising regularly, this balance returned.

He then conducted a similar study by moving blue-collar workers to sedentary desk jobs. The results were just what he expected. They ate more and gained weight. Once they returned to manual work, they ate less and lost the weight.[7]

There appears to be some kind of balance between how much we eat and how many calories we burn up. An adequate amount of exercise will help us lose weight, not simply because we are burning up calories, but because proper exercise helps maintain that delicate balance in our systems.

The everyday changes are the ones that will make the differences for us. Playing touch football once a year or bowling once a month will not have much effect. But daily exercise will make the difference. For instance, consider taking the stairs to the fourth floor four times a day instead of the elevator. Walk sometimes instead of driving. Stand instead of sitting. It's important to incorporate the more active ways of doing things into our day-to-day lives.

We live in a convenient society, a society in which we are surrounded by machinery and appliances designed to make our lives easier. But these conveniences contribute to our weight problems.

Your goal should be to get into the habit of choosing the more active way of doing things. No matter how unathletic you have been in the past, start thinking of yourself as an active, athletic person, quick to get up and get going. Perhaps you drive wherever you go, ride in the golf cart rather than walk, take the more lazy, passive way of doing things. Put that behind you and begin to think of yourself as active and athletic, no matter how far from reality that image of yourself may seem.

Look for ways in your life to increase the amount of daily exercise that you are getting, even if only in small ways. You may decide to park ten spaces further from the store than you usually do. Or you may choose the stairs rather than the escalator. Activities like this are not going to burn up that many calories, but they will help you begin thinking differently about yourself. As you make these small changes, you will gain confidence that will give you incentive to look for other ways to be active.

You may want to consider cutting down from three to only one telephone in the house. It's excellent exercise to run upstairs or downstairs to answer the phone. Or you may want to plant your own vegetable garden. Avoid looking for the easy, automated way of doing things. One or two appliances do not make that much difference, but several can cut down on the calories you would otherwise burn up. Decide, on occasion, not to use the remote-control television switch, electric knife, electric toothbrush, snow blower, or riding lawnmower.

Because we live in such a highly automated society, we have to engage in such activities as running in circles around a track that goes nowhere. Otherwise we will not get enough exercise to keep our bodies healthy and well-functioning.

Several years ago I was visiting some good friends who own a large corn and soybean farm. Mr. Brown, the farmer, watched me in amazement as I went through my daily exercise routine of toe-touches, jumping jacks, sit-ups, and jogging. Able to contain himself no longer, he remarked with a chuckle, "Why don't you just work?"

Of course it must have seemed silly to a hardworking man like Mr. Brown to see a city slicker like myself wasting all that energy. Even so, I have come to accept the fact that, given my lifestyle, I need this kind of exercise. I do not live on a farm, where there are plenty of opportunities for hard manual labor. To be healthy and to keep my weight down, I need to engage in some seemingly useless activities, like jumping in the air and running around the block.

Aerobic Exercise

Aerobic simply means "with oxygen." In addition to choosing to be more active in your day-to-day life, you should also begin to incorporate some type of aerobic exercise into your schedule.

Some years ago I was vacationing with my mother. She would get up every morning as I lay in bed and perform her daily exercise routine. Later in the day as we hiked in the mountains, I would be amazed to find her endurance much greater than mine. After that vacation, I decided it was high time I started a regular exercise program.

A friend and I agreed to exercise together five days a week. We did that for a full year, with only a few misses. Later, we started jogging regularly, and I have been jogging about six miles a week for the last two and a half years. I now think of myself as a fairly athletic person. Granted, I will probably never win the Boston Marathon, but my endurance is greater than ever before for such activities as hiking, living life, and serving God.

Three factors were essential to the success of my exercise program. One factor was that I had lost the weight I needed to. I felt more comfortable exercising and more confident that I could succeed at it. The second factor was my agreement to exercise with an equally motivated friend. The third consisted of my decision to make exercise a regular part of my schedule. Exercise was not an extra, tacked on to the end of the day, but a regular part of my morning routine.

Jogging has served as an enjoyable form of exercise for me. But not everyone takes to it as I did. Some people can think of nothing worse. If you do not like jogging, find some other kind of exercise. Walking can be great exercise. Riding an exercycle or bicycle, swimming, and jumping rope are all excellent means of exercise.

Choose exercises that use the large muscles, like the leg muscles. Such exercises burn up more calories than those using smaller muscles, like the arms. Exercises that require you to carry your own weight use more calories. Jogging, running, and jumping rope, will burn up more calories than swimming or bike riding. The latter are good exercises, but they do not take as many calories to perform. At the end of this chapter is a list of exercises and the corresponding number of calories burned up while you do them.

Do I Have to Exercise to Lose Weight?

The answer is no. You will lose weight simply by eating fewer calories than you use. Exercise may help you lose weight a bit faster, but it is often better to wait on an exercise program until you have lost some of your initial weight and gained some confidence.

One of my patients never exercised. If she visited a friend a block away, she would drive. If she wanted to go to two stores in the same shopping center, she would drive to the first one, park, shop, and then return to the car and drive to the other one. She was so overweight and out of shape that any amount of exercise left her breathless. When she started to lose weight, I never even mentioned exercise. It would have been too much for her. But after she had lost about fifty pounds, she began a simple exercise program that consisted of taking short walks. Before long she was taking longer walks and even walking the two miles to her appointment with me.

Exercise will not only help you lose weight, it will help you maintain your weight loss. And it offers many other benefits as well: greater endurance, improved self-image, a stronger cardiovascular system, and stronger muscles that will serve you better.

Getting Started

Begin with very small steps. Be realistic. You might start by simply walking to the mailbox and back. Or you might decide to walk around the block once. Start with an activity that is easy to accomplish. Having taken the first, small step you will have greater confidence when it comes to taking the second, larger step. If you start with an overwhelming goal, perhaps deciding to run two miles four times a week, you will probably become so tired and sore that you will want to abandon your exercise program for good.

Try to set up your exercise program with a friend, or perhaps with your spouse. A short walk after dinner or a jog as soon as the children are off to school might be just the right thing. Find a partner who is also interested in starting an exercise program, someone at about the same level of fitness that you are. Nothing is more discouraging than jogging with someone who can run circles around you or swimming with someone who can go two laps to your one.

Keep at It

Whenever you want to increase the frequency of an activity, schedule it before, rather than after, an already frequent activity. For instance, say that you are trying to get into the habit of making your bed in the morning. You decide that you will not eat breakfast until the bed is made. Your resolve will probably work. But would it have worked if you had decided to make the bed only after you had eaten? Probably not. Likewise, plan your exercise time before, rather than after, an already frequent activity. For example, you decide to exercise with a brisk walk in the evening. Your habit is to have a cup of coffee after dinner. You could decide to drink your coffee only after your walk.

One morning the alarm rang, and I found myself lying in bed, thinking, "Do I feel like running today?" Before I could answer, I thought to myself, "Wait a minute. It doesn't matter whether I *feel* like it or not. Today is my day to run and I am going to do it." If I asked myself if I *felt* like running, I would probably run only rarely.

You don't make other decisions based on how you feel. You work every day regardless of how you feel about it. You cook dinner whether or not you feel like it. By the same token, you should exercise regardless of whether you feel like it. Don't even ask yourself that question. You have set out a plan or a program for yourself, and you are going to stick to it. The question of whether you feel like it is irrelevant. Just get out there and do it.

Another way to get started is to take a class. Take a tennis class, an aerobics dance class, a swimming class. It helps to take a class that meets two or three times a week. That way, you will be more likely to report regularly to class and participate in the exercise. If you paid for a class that meets Tuesday and Thursday nights at 6:45, you will probably attend. However, if you simply promise yourself to go to the pool on Monday nights without making a commitment to a class or a friend, you will be much less likely to do it.

Look around your area for what is available. You need not be embarrassed to take a class. Chances are that the other members of the class will be people just like you. They are not champion athletes, just beginners. You will probably find that many of them are people who are or were overweight. Like you, they want to become more active to stay in shape.

Check the local YMCA, YWCA, or recreation department for a listing of available classes. Promise yourself that you will go to the class at least two or three times. A decision like that can help you conquer any fear you might have about the class. If you can get yourself to go the first time, you will probably go back. If you are terribly uncomfortable, if the class does not meet your needs, or if it is not at all what you had in mind, then you can quit. No one will force you to continue. But promise yourself that you will give it a try.

Buy some good equipment and suitable clothing. You will feel more at ease on the tennis court in the appropriate clothing. And you will enjoy jogging, running, or walking more if you have some good shoes. Resist the temptation to wear that old pair of baggy shorts that belong in the trash bin or that swimsuit that you have worn for the last ten years. Invest in sports clothes that are attractive and comfortable.

You need not be afraid of getting sweaty and dirty. If you exercise energetically you probably will perspire. If you have a set of clothes that are strictly for exercise, you will not mind getting them dirty. A shower and change after your exercise period will leave you feeling invigorated and refreshed. For many people, a hot shower and fresh clothes mark the high point of their exercise routine. They are a reward for hard work.

Be sure to choose the right time for starting your exercise program. Begin with small steps. Find a friend to join you. Get the right kind of clothing and equipment. Regular exercise will open up a whole new aspect of life to you. You probably will have some fears about it, but go ahead and try it. You may be surprised by what you discover.

Week Eight Assignment:

Keep an exercise diary. This can be part of your food diary or you can use a separate page for it. Every day record your increased activity. Use the one that follows as an example.

Figure 7
Exercise Diary—Sample

Date	Exercise
6/26	Ran two miles Parked car at far end of lot and walked to store
6/27	Took stairs instead of the elevator
6/28	Worked in garden for two hours
6/29	Ran two miles
6/30	Went swimming for fifteen minutes Took the dog for a five-minute walk
7/1	Golfed a nine-hole course
7/2	Took a ten-minute walk

The chart on the facing page indicates calorie expenditures for common activities. It was prepared by Robert E. Johnson, M.D., Ph.D., and colleagues, Department of Physiology and Biophysics, University of Illinois, August 1967. Reprinted from "Exercise and Weight Control," President's Council on Physical Fitness and Sports (Washington, D.C.: U.S. Government Printing Ofc., 1980).

Figure 8

Energy Expenditure by a 150 Pound Person in Various Activities*

Activity	Calories Per Hour
A. Rest and Light Activity	**50-200**
Lying down or sleeping	80
Sitting	100
Driving an automobile	120
Standing	140
Domestic work	180
B. Moderate Activity	**200-350**
Bicycling (5½ mph)	210
Walking (2½ mph)	210
Gardening	220
Canoeing (2½ mph)	230
Golf	250
Lawn mowing (power mower)	250
Bowling	270
Lawn mowing (hand mower)	270
Fencing	300
Rowboating (2½ mph)	300
Swimming (¼ mph)	300
Walking (3¾ mph)	300
Badminton	350
Horseback riding (trotting)	350
Square dancing	350
Volleyball	350
Roller skating	350
C. Vigorous Activity	**over 350**
Table tennis	360
Ditch digging (hand shovel)	400
Ice skating (10 mph)	400
Wood chopping or sawing	400
Tennis	420
Water skiing	480
Hill climbing (100 ft. per hr.)	490
Skiing (10 mph)	600
Squash and handball	600
Cycling (13 mph)	660
Scull rowing (race)	840
Running (10 mph)	900

*The standards represent a compromise between those proposed by the British Medical Association (1950), Christensen (1953), and Wells, Balke, and Van Fossan (1956). Where available, actual measured values have been used; for other values a "best guess" was made.

NINE

Reward for a Job Well-Done

ONE OF THE REASONS that weight problems are so difficult to control is that eating is a self-reinforcing activity. When you are face-to-face with a cookie, eating is the action that will immediately reinforce you. The prospect of a thin and healthy body two or three months from now is not particularly reinforcing at the moment the impulse strikes. However, if someone offered you $10 not to eat the cookie you were just then reaching for, my bet is that you wouldn't eat it. The $10 bill would reinforce your good choice.

Since no one is running around with $10 bills to hand out, you will need some other kind of reward system. The best one I know of is called a token reinforcement system. Under this system you earn tokens for good behavior, and these tokens in turn earn you particular rewards.

Do not reward yourself simply for weight loss. Your weight can be very unpredictable. Instead, reward yourself for specific behavior changes, like sitting at your designated eating place consistently. The idea is to give yourself points, or tokens, for certain behaviors. Later, you will redeem these points for predetermined rewards. You can use an old checkbook register to keep track of your points. When you earn points, enter a deposit in your checkbook. When you give yourself a reward, make a withdrawal from your checkbook. Refer to the token reward chart at the end of the chapter for how many points to award yourself for certain kinds of behavior.

Another system is based on contingent rewards. In other words, collecting a particular reward is contingent on a particular behavior. For instance, you tell yourself that you can watch your favorite television show tonight if you sit at your eating place consistently today. You can involve another person in the reward, but do it carefully. You want to avoid feeling pressured. For instance, you could agree with a close friend to go to a movie Saturday night if you stick to your diet this week. If you stray from the diet, then say goodbye to the movie.

You can also give yourself small, more immediate rewards. For instance, say that you have handled a difficult food situation at work well. It is perfectly legitimate to buy yourself some diet pop on your way home as a small reward. Sometimes it is enough of a reward to simply tell yourself that you did a good job. But do reward yourself. Losing weight is not easy, and you need positive reinforcement to succeed. You can no longer depend on food as a reward, but you still need to reinforce good behavior.

Be creative when it comes to looking for ways to celebrate and to reward yourself and others. Perhaps one of your co-workers just got a promotion. In the past you would have brought in donuts to celebrate. This time, try something that has nothing to do with food. Buy him a small gift, something related to his favorite hobby, or tickets to a play. Such gifts often take a bit more thought, but they are always appreciated, and they keep you out of trouble.

When you feel in need of a reward, choose a non-food treat. Buy a new book, a favorite magazine, a new plant, or something else that appeals to you. But never resort to food. People with weight problems often fail to allow themselves any pleasures in life. They don't even really allow themselves food. But food is the one treat they can get their hands on. Consequently, they try to meet much of their need for pleasure and reward through food.

Experiment with different kinds of rewards. Try the token reinforcement system and see if it helps you. Try using contingent rewards and spontaneous rewards as well. It's fine to reward yourself for weight loss after a while, perhaps after you have lost twenty pounds. It helps to congratulate yourself for a job well done. Or you may want to wait until you reach your goal weight. I frequently suggest that my patients buy some new clothing after a significant weight loss, even though they have not yet reached their goal. They are reinforced for good behavior, and they feel good in the new clothes. They usually get more compliments and are generally reinforced for all the hard work they have done.

Watching the numbers on the scale go down every week is reinforcing in itself. For some people that is enough of a reward to maintain their motivation. Your reward may come from knowing that you are gaining control over your eating behavior. As Christians, a certain amount of our reward will also come from the knowledge that we are gaining greater patience, perseverance, and maturity. That, in itself, makes it worth the struggle.

If you find the reward system helpful, use it until the new behaviors become firmly established, and then gradually wean yourself from the rewards. The purpose of using reinforcers is to help yourself begin new habits. But, ultimately, you should not have to reward yourself for every good behavior.

Losing weight is not easy. It takes a lot of hard work. But in the end, you will feel better physically, and you will feel better about yourself for having lost the weight. Undoubtedly, there will be many times when you will prefer to give up. But resist the temptation. If you quit, you will never experience the fruit of all your work. Stay with it. You won't regret it.

Week Nine Assignment:

1. Make a token reward chart.
   —List different behaviors that you want to work on, and indicate their worth in points.
   —List various rewards, some small and some large,

and indicate how many points are needed to earn
them.
2. Using an old checkbook register or a chart made to
resemble one, keep track of your behaviors and the
points earned. Claim your rewards as you earn them and
deduct the points from your balance.

Figure 9
Token Reward Chart—Sample

Behavior	Points
Staying on diet and weighing and measuring food for one day	1 point
Keeping food diary for one day	1
Sitting at eating place consistently for one day	1
Eating slowly at all meals for one day	1
Using a two-minute break at every meal	1
Putting food out of sight for one day	1
Running one mile	1
two miles	1
three miles	1

Possible Rewards	Total Points Needed
Tickets to a concert	10 points
One hour in library for pleasure reading	10
A drive in the country	10
Buy myself a magazine	15
Buy myself a book	20
Lunch out with a friend	20
New piece of clothing worth $20	50
New rod and reel	75

Figure 10
Reward Account—Sample

Date	Behavior or Reward	Points Deposited	Points Withdrawn	Balance
5/1	Stayed on diet	1		1
5/1	Eating place	1		2
5/1	Ran 3 miles	3		5
5/2	Diet, eating place	2		7
5/3	Diet, eating place	2		9
5/3	Ran 3 miles	3		12
5/4	Bought magazine		10	2

Planning Puts You in Control

RECENTLY, I ATTENDED a party with a group of friends. When dessert was offered, one of the women—a rather thin, attractive person—turned it down. When someone asked why, she responded that she was going out to dinner on Saturday and planned to eat dessert then, so she wasn't going to have it now. The party was on a Tuesday night. This woman, who appeared to be "naturally" thin, seemed to have a built-in ability to plan ahead. Though it was only Tuesday night, she had already thought ahead and decided to have dessert on Saturday and to forgo it the rest of the week.

Many thin people do this naturally. They think ahead and make decisions about the food they plan to eat or not eat. The overweight person is less likely to think ahead even one evening, much less to the end of the week. Planning ahead simply involves thinking about food before you actually come face-to-face with it. If you have planned ahead, you are much more likely to stay on your diet. You have already decided how to relate to particular situations.

Let's say that you are going to a party Friday night. You have had a very busy day, and you have not thought much about the party. You eat hastily and finally arrive at the party about 9:00. As soon as you walk in you notice a table laden with an interesting variety of snacks, hors d'oeuvres, and desserts. Suddenly, you are faced with a decision you had not anticipated. Chances are you will not keep to your diet.

Now consider another situation. You plan to attend a wedding reception on Saturday afternoon. You have been keeping your food diary, planning ahead, and doing well on your diet. You do not want the reception to be an excuse to go off your diet. To prepare yourself, you talk with the bride's sister and find out what the menu will be. Once you know the menu, you decide what you will eat and drink. You even imagine yourself selecting certain foods and politely refusing others. You are comfortable and confident about your decision. Under such circumstances, chances are you will do exactly as you planned. You are ready for the reception. The food will not take you by surprise.

Do your planning on paper, first a day at a time and later a week at a time. Sit down and plan the next twenty-four hours. Think about the different times that you will be eating and write down the time and exactly what you plan to eat.

7:30 A.M.	1 cup corn flakes 1 cup skim milk ½ cup orange juice coffee, black
12:30 P.M.	2 oz. cheese 5 saltines lettuce salad sliced tomato 1 tablespoon low-calorie dressing 1 medium peach iced tea
3:30 P.M.	1 small apple coffee, black
6:30 P.M.	4 oz. broiled fish ½ cup cooked rice ½ cup cooked carrots ½ cup green beans

lettuce salad with mushrooms
1 tablespoon low-calorie dressing
¼ cantaloupe

9:00 P.M.   ½ cup ice milk

With the whole day planned, you are much more likely to follow your diet.

This week, plan ahead twenty-four hours at a time. Set aside a certain time of the day for your planning. You may want to do it in the morning after breakfast, while you are still drinking your coffee. Sketch out on paper what you will be eating for the next twenty-four hours. Include your snacks as well as your meals. If there are any special occasions coming up, plan those. As you plan, picture the different settings you will be in. Imagine yourself eating slowly, having a good time, feeling proud that you have handled the occasion so well. All of this will greatly increase your chances of success.

Eventually, you will be able to do this mentally. It will be second nature to think ahead about where you will be and what you will be eating. Continue to write your plans on paper until you think that you can do it mentally. Remember that a well-planned, well-functioning schedule can bring peace and order to your life, and ease and success to your diet.

In my years as a nurse, I have been impressed with the regular, methodical schedules of many of my elderly patients. It is not uncommon to hear one of them say, "Every night at 9:00, I have a glass of warm milk and go to bed. I get up at 5:30 A.M. and have my oatmeal and apple juice." The rest of their day is characterized by a similar kind of regularity.

People devise and use a regular, systematic schedule because it works. After years of experience, they have found that it brings peace and personal order into their lives.

Youth tends to value spontaneity. It's more fun and exciting. "Let's stay up and watch the late movie." No matter that you get to bed at 3:00 A.M. and drag yourself through the next day. As we mature, we recognize that youthful spontaneity often has painful consequences. As a result, we value the peace and stability that comes from having a regular schedule. Gone are the days when we are tempted by an intriguing ad for the late show.

If your life is impulsive and spontaneous, then your eating will be impulsive and spontaneous. Your goal should be to live according to a sane, rational, mature plan. Your eating habits should reflect the same basic order as the rest of your life. You get up in the morning in time to go to work or get the kids off to school. You don't wait until you feel like getting up. Similarly, you eat in order to meet your nutritional needs, not in order to satisfy your impulses.

Vacations

Plan your vacations the same way you would your day-to-day life. Your vacation does not need to be rigorous and tightly scheduled. But do plan for it. Plan your mealtime, bedtime, and rising time. Plan what you will be eating and what you will be doing.

If you decide to do your own cooking on vacation, at a cottage or camp, then plan a menu for the entire time. But plan special things that you would not ordinarily have, maybe steaks and fresh fish, special fruits and vegetables. Do your grocery shopping according to your menu. Bring along a good supply of the kinds of foods that will support your diet.

Menu Planning and Grocery Shopping

Once every two weeks I sit down with a cup of coffee, a calendar, and a few cookbooks to plan dinner meals for the upcoming two weeks. I try to consider the nights we will have guests and the nights when I will want to make a quick, easy supper. Then I take out a copy of what I call my master marketing list. This itemizes everything I normally buy in the grocery store, listed in the order in which the items are found in the store that I shop at regularly. I have enough copies made to last a year.

I review the menu and mark off the list those ingredients that I will need for various meals. Then I go back over the grocery list and check off all the other things I will need—cereal and juice for breakfast, food for lunches, paper goods, and so on. The whole process takes less than an hour and saves several hours, not to mention headaches, during the next week.

Use this plan or devise your own but do figure out a way to plan your menus and to keep your trips to the grocery at a minimum. Remember, every time you go to the store, you are exposing yourself to that many more food cues.

Week Ten Assignment:

1. Plan what you will eat in the next twenty-four hours, writing down in your food diary what you plan to eat at what time.
2. Plan menus for your main meals for one week at a time.

Master Marketing List

Produce	Cans and Boxes	Rx
lettuce	pineapple	wetting solution
carrots	applesauce	soaking solution
apples	lemon juice	Crest
celery	tomatoes	shampoo
onions	tomato sauce	creme rinse
cabbage	tomato paste	Ban
bananas	ketchup	Old Spice
grapefruit	mustard	hair spray
mushrooms	Worchestershire	razor blades
grapes	sauce	Metamucil
potatoes	vinegar	
peppers	Heinz 57	

tomatoes
other:

Bread

hotdog buns
hamburger buns
sandwich bread
rye bread
thin bread

Crackers/Cookies

club crackers
other:

Dairy

eggs
milk
tortillas
margarine
English muffins
cheese
  cheddar
  Swiss
  slices
  other:

Frozen

orange juice
lemonade
bread
peas
broccoli
spinach
mixed vegetables

pickles
relish
peanut butter
jelly
salad dressing
tuna
rice
macaroni and cheese
spaghetti
macaroni
oatmeal
cold cereal
soups
syrup
croutons
other:

Mexican

taco shells
green chilis
taco sauce

Meats

ground beef
pot roast
cube steak

Baking

powdered milk
flour
sugar-white
sugar-brown
salt
cornstarch
oil
spices:

Paper

toilet paper
Kleenex
paper towels
napkins
garbage bags
  kitchen
garbage bags
  30 gal.
Handiwrap
foil
lunch bags
sandwich bags
freezer bags
paper plates
styrofoam cups
light bulbs
other:

Soaps

Jergens
Pledge
Era
Cheer
bleach
cleanser
dish detergent
spray sizing
Windex
other:

Lunch Meats

bacon
ham
braunschweiger
bologna
other:

green beans
  French cut
cauliflower
brussel sprouts
squash
carrots
hash browns
T.V. dinners

Coffee

ground coffee
instant coffee
Brim
tea bags
iced tea mix
lemonade mix
coffee filters

Treats

potato chips
Weight Watcher's
  ice cream
ice milk

ELEVEN

Feelings and Food
What Is the Connection?

F ROM THE TIME we are very young, we learn to cope with our feelings by eating. Little Johnny falls and scrapes his knee. Mom cleans and bandages it and then soothes Johnny by giving him a candy bar. It works. He is happy and soon forgets about his scraped knee. But what is really happening? Johnny is learning that the way to cope with unhappiness is by eating nice treats.

Years later, he still handles life's ups and downs the same way. Every time he becomes lonely or depressed, he turns to food to help him cope. Such behavior is not the worst response to hardship, but it does have its problems. In order to lose weight and keep it off, Johnny will need to learn a new and more constructive way to handle his feelings.

All of us need comfort and consolation in life, but not from food. As Christians, we know that the Lord wants to be our comfort and consolation. If we run to food every time we have a need, we prevent him from coming into our hearts to fill that need. We have taken care of the problem ourselves. We should be willing to live with the need or hurt for a time, whether it means waiting a few minutes, hours, or even days, until the Lord shows us his way of dealing with it.

Sometimes comfort will come directly from God. Go before him in a quiet, private place and allow him to speak to you. Read scripture or some other spiritual book if you think that will help.

God may use what you are reading as a vehicle for communicating with you, or he may speak to you directly, giving you consolation, new hope, and perspective on the difficulty you are having. He may offer you support and insight through a friend that you can confide in. But if you cope with the need in your own way, by reaching for something to eat, you will probably never rely on the Lord to meet your need.

We use food in this way because it often does work. If you are depressed and eat something you like, it may seem to help, if only momentarily. It may soothe you a bit and allow you to push ahead. Almost everyone does this once in a while. But the problem is that most overweight people do it all the time. Every time they become depressed, angry, or anxious they eat.

Depression

Carolyn told me that she had been depressed as far back as she could remember. As a child she used to take long walks alone, letting depression engulf her. In college, she actually enjoyed sitting in a dark room reading by the light of a single candle or writing melancholy poetry. She never tried to deal with her depression. To her it was just life, and life was depressing.

After she committed her life to the Lord, she expected the depression to disappear. But she continued to experience it daily. For years, she woke up feeling depressed and heavy, not wanting or daring to face the day. After a while she learned to cope with the depression by eating. Whenever she felt depressed, she would look for something to eat. Her friends never knew of her problem. She hid it fairly well and seemed to enjoy life, even though she was bitterly depressed.

The turning point came when she began to understand that self-pity was at the root of her depression. She realized that self-pity is wrong and that it requires repentance. She began to ask God to forgive her for it. Every time she felt a twinge of depression, she would ask why she was feeling sorry for herself.

Sometimes she needed to dig deep, but she always found the reason. Even after she identified the reason, she would sometimes have to struggle to let go of the self-pity. There were too many "good" reasons to feel sorry for herself. But she knew that the longer she clung to the self-pity, the longer her depression would last.

Her fight against self-pity succeeded, and the depression lifted completely. That was several years ago. Since then, she says, she has had perhaps ten days of depression. Before that she had hardly spent ten days without it. This simple but profound truth set her free from a problem that had plagued her for years.

Depression used to make Carolyn overeat, but not anymore. She learned to deal with the overeating and also with the depression. To maintain her weight she still has to be faithful to her diet, using all the behavioral techniques she has learned, but at least she no longer needs to fight depression and its effects on her eating habits.

Anger

Are you the kind of person who never gets angry? Are you always cool, calm, and collected, no matter what? Do people ever tell you that they are amazed because you never seem to let things bother you? You never blow up.

Look again. Is anger hidden under that calm exterior? Are you using food to keep yourself calm? If you are using food in this way, you may not even be aware of the anger.

Consider this sequence of events. You argue with a co-worker, but you handle the disagreement calmly. Immediately afterwards you head for the vending machines. You have been doing well on your diet for weeks. All of a sudden you find yourself with a candy bar in hand. What are you doing? Most probably you are responding according to an old pattern, quietly repressing the anger inside of you. As a matter of fact, your technique works. You eat the candy bar and are able to go back to work. The only person you are upset with is yourself for eating the candy. Though it can work, eating to control your anger does nothing for you in the long run and only makes your weight problem worse.

The first step in dealing with anger is to recognize it. Ask yourself why you want to eat. What just happened? Why are you standing at the ice-cream counter when you have stuck to your diet for weeks? Are you angry with something or someone? Recognize the anger. Put your finger on exactly what caused it.

Second, formulate a plan. Ask yourself how you can deal constructively with the anger. Brainstorm. Consider every possible way to handle the situation that has made you angry. Learn to deal with conflict. Don't be afraid of it. It may even help you face it better if you imagine the worst thing that could happen.

Anger is not wrong in itself. It is a feeling. But it is one that our society teaches us to repress, to keep quiet. We learn that it is not appropriate to scream and yell and slam doors, but we do not learn how to express anger righteously and assertively. And there are times when we ought to express it. Instead, we repress it by eating.

Make a decision about how you are going to handle your anger. Perhaps you should go to the person who provoked you and talk the situation through. Maybe you need to admit your pride and self-righteousness and ask the Lord to help you approach the situation with patience and love. Dealing with anger may mean letting go of resentment and learning to view a particular situation from a fresh perspective.

Perhaps you need to learn how to be more assertive. If you are properly assertive, you will be able to avoid many situations that could lead to anger and the consequent need to repress it by eating. Assertiveness is not the same as aggressiveness. It does not mean always getting your own way or bossing others around. It simply means making your needs, opinions, or preferences known in a non-defensive, straightforward manner. If you are properly assertive, you will not threaten the other person, but enable him to see your point and encourage him to respond positively rather than angrily or aggressively.

Quite commonly, overweight people lack assertiveness. When asked their preference about something, they may respond that they have no preference when in fact they do. Consequently, when a decision has been made that makes them unhappy, they have to find some way to deal with it. Instead of saying anything, they look for something to eat in order to repress their anger.

Let's say that Joe is waiting at the counter at the hardware store when another man cuts in front of him. He could decide to let it go and say nothing. After all, he is not in a hurry and this other fellow is obviously in a big rush. It would be perfectly fine for him to decide not to make an issue of it. But it would also be fine for Joe to say to the man or the clerk, "Excuse me, but I believe I was next in line." That is an example of being assertive.

If Joe is angry that the man cut in front of him, but says nothing, he will leave the store angry, and he may stop to get something to eat on his way home simply to repress his anger.

Anxiety

We use food to deal with anxiety in much the same way that we use it to deal with anger. We eat to calm us down and to help us cope with anxiety. As with anger, it does not really make the anxiety go away, but it does offer a temporary remedy. But, once again, this remedy comes at great cost to ourselves. How can we deal with anxiety without eating?

First of all, learn to recognize anxiety. You cannot deal with it effectively unless you can identify what is going on. A person who is overweight will often use food to cope with the stresses of life. Losing weight and keeping it off means learning new ways of dealing with stress.

I remember coming home from work once and hearing that my roommate's father had died. I was shocked and felt sad for her family. At the same time, I remember a thought that crossed my mind. "I can't stay on my diet. Sharon's father died. I'll just have to eat whatever the family brings over." Before that I had been doing very well. The thought made absolutely no sense. I could have just as easily eaten a low-calorie dinner as a high-calorie one. But because of my anxiety, I made a poor decision.

Second, write out a plan. Sit down with pencil and paper and make a simple plan about how you are going to deal with the situation that is causing your anxiety. Break your plan into manageable parts. Take it one day at a time or even one hour at a time. It does no good to worry about next week or next year. God is not giving you the grace right now for tomorrow, for next week, or next year. He is giving you what you need for today, and that is all.

Your anxiety may often be focused on your diet. You might find yourself thinking, "I can't stay on this diet forever"; "I just don't know how I'm going to handle Christmas"; "I'll never lose all this weight." This kind of thinking will make you reach for the nearest cookie or candy bar. It almost insures defeat. Don't allow yourself to think this way. You only need to get through this next hour and this next day. That is all the Lord is giving you grace for. Worry about tomorrow when tomorrow comes. If your mind starts to race ahead, pull it back. You can make it through the next hour, and that is all you need to be concerned about.

Consider Sam's experience. He had been asked to give a presentation for his company. It was just the kind of request that made him nervous. As the day for the presentation drew near, his anxiety increased and so did his desire to eat. He decided to formulate a plan to overcome his temptation. This was it:

1. Talk to a co-worker tomorrow about the presentation and about his anxiety in order to receive some support and reassurance.

2. State the truth to himself. "I have done things like this before, and I can do it again. I probably will not faint. My boss believes I can do it or he would not have asked me."

3. Continue his regular exercise routine as a way to relieve the anxiety.

4. Bring his mind back to thinking only about the next hour rather than letting it race ahead to the presentation.

5. Accept the fact that some degree of tension is normal and can actually help motivate people to accomplish a difficult task.

Sam's plan worked, and he actually lost weight the week before the presentation!

Self-Esteem

Low self-esteem is a frequent factor in weight problems, particularly among women. When we feel bad about ourselves we can tend to overeat, and the more we overeat the worse we feel about ourselves. It's the classic vicious circle. As Christians, our self-esteem comes from our identity as sons and daughters of the Father, not from how successful or how thin we are.

It is just as wrong to hate yourself as it is to hate your neighbor. Regardless of how many good reasons you may think you have, it is still wrong to hate, judge, or condemn yourself. If you have been doing this, then you need to go before the Lord and repent, asking his forgiveness. Decide that you are going to accept yourself and make the best of who you are and the gifts you have.

A fat self-image is another false impression that the Lord can heal. A person with a "fat self-image" thinks of himself as fat no matter what. He cannot imagine himself as thin or as capable of becoming thin. "But," you might object, "I *am* fat. I have always been fat and always will be. Nothing I can do will ever change that." Whatever your objections, it simply is not true that you have no choice but to be overweight. Ask God to change that image and to give you new hope.

Guilt

Anyone with a weight problem has probably experienced some amount of guilt about it. When you feel guilty, you have a sense that you have done something wrong, that you are being judged. Along with guilt feelings can come self-condemnation, lack of self-esteem, and a feeling that others, including the Lord, are judging and condemning you. Guilt can sometimes be good, as when it causes you to repent of sin. But when it is connected with food and weight, it often comes either from the flesh or from the evil one.

Certain kinds of guilt can be vague and difficult to deal with. You might feel that you did something terribly wrong, but you are not sure how to set it right or even if you can set it right. You are convinced that anyone who knew your fault would judge and condemn you for it.

Mary was doing well on her diet until she woke up one day feeling tired and irritable. She ate her regular breakfast and dressed for work. While waiting for her ride, she wandered into the kitchen looking for something to eat. She was standing at the counter nibbling on something when she heard a knock on the door. Her car pool had arrived.

She felt awful. "If they knew what I was doing," she thought, "they would think I was terrible. I am so undisciplined that I can't even control the way I eat." By the time she reached the car, she was quiet and reserved, fearful of looking at or talking to anyone lest she meet with knowing and judgmental stares. Of course her companions had no idea what she had been doing. And they probably couldn't have cared less about it had they known.

This incident set up a downward spiral for Mary's day. She became discouraged and depressed. Everything she did was colored by a vague sense of guilt. This only set her up for eating more than she should have the rest of the day. Afterwards, she felt guilty, self-pitying, and ready to give up on her diet.

Mary's nibbling in the kitchen was a mistake, but it did not constitute serious wrongdoing. Yes, she was on a diet and she should not have eaten. But she needed to put her mistake behind her and get on with her day. No one was judging her. Quite likely, she will make similar errors in the future. When she does, she will have to guard against magnifying them out of all proportion to reality.

If you eat something that is not on your diet, you probably are not guilty of wrongdoing. But it is certainly wrong to let yourself become trapped by guilt, self-pity, and despair. That is what you should repent for. If you go off your diet, okay. Get right back on. Avoid using one failure as an opportunity to wallow in self-pity and hopelessness. If you do, you will only eat something else and feel even guiltier as a result. Get up and keep going. You can do it.

Inner Healing

Inner healing, the healing of emotional, mental, and spiritual difficulties from the past, probably is not *the* answer to your weight problem. It can play a part, of course, but it usually does not supply the whole remedy. I used to think that once God had healed enough hurts from the past I would magically lose weight. The years went by. I grew in Christian maturity. My life was in good basic order. The Lord did heal many hurts from my past. But I was still overweight.

Finally, I realized that I needed to go on a diet to lose the weight. In the course of my efforts, I learned about many of the behavioral techniques that I have already explained in this book. Losing weight involved more than just being "whole" spiritually; it involved a change in my lifestyle and habits.

Of course inner healing can play a role in the weight-losing process. It may be appropriate to pray for inner healing at the beginning of your diet or even after you are well on your way to losing the extra weight. You could ask a friend, counselor, or pastor to pray with you, to ask the Lord to heal any emotional difficulties that may have contributed to your weight problem.

You Are Not a Hopeless Case

Just because you experience one failure or, for that matter, a series of failures does not mean that you are a hopeless case. You are not. If you have given in to self-pity, repent for it. You *will* be a hopeless case if you sit there and stew, letting yourself be swallowed up in your thoughts. The choice is yours. It may not be easy, but you can refuse to feel sorry for yourself.

Set realistic goals. If you are a thirty-five-year-old woman, 5'6" tall, and weigh in at 175 pounds, it probably is not realistic to expect yourself to slim down to the 115 pounds you weighed in high school. You are a grown woman now. Set a more realistic goal.

Whenever you set unrealistic goals for yourself, you set yourself up for failure. It is far better to embark on a course that will end in victory. Don't make it as hard as possible to succeed. Make it as easy as you can.

Week Eleven Assignment:

Keep a log of your negative feelings and how you respond to them. Write down your typical responses to depression, fatigue, anxiety, anger, and so on. Choose one feeling to work on this week. Ask the Lord to show you how to deal with it. It may be something as simple as taking a nap or calling a friend just to chat. Or perhaps you need to repent to the Lord and others for feeling sorry for yourself or for being irritable.

Resist becoming discouraged if you fail to make the right choice every time. Remember, you are trying to change a long-standing way of responding to certain feelings. Be patient with yourself. But keep trying. And avoid the tendency to become overly introspective. It is good to understand how your emotions work, but you should not scrutinize them to the point that you are always thinking about how you feel.

TWELVE

Negative Thinking

JOHN JUST HUNG UP the phone. The company he was trying to recruit as a client for the past six weeks just turned him down. He is tired. The next thing he knows, he is standing at the candy machine, three candy bars in hand.

Not five minutes after the last bite of candy is consumed, the self-condemnation begins. He has been dieting for a month now and has lost twelve pounds, but this incident marks failure. It just proves he is incapable of losing weight. He has always turned to food in the past and always will. Sure, he can try to change, but he will never really be successful. Thoroughly discouraged, he gives up on the diet for now. It is just too hard.

John is not listening to truth but to a lie. And because he is putting his faith in a lie, he is going to be defeated. If he hangs onto self-doubt and self-criticism and the sure doom of failure, that is exactly what he is going to get.

How can you avoid the trap John fell into?

First, learn to recognize lies and self-defeating, negative thoughts for what they are. Is that kind of thing from God? Is this the way he would want you to think about yourself? Definitely not.

Second, rebuke the lie. Take authority over what is going on in your mind. Never let those kind of thoughts stay. Your mind belongs to you, and you have control over what stays in it. Avoid entertaining negative, self-condemning thoughts. Such thoughts are self-defeating, and it is wrong to harbor them. If you have been indulging in them, repent and turn away from them.

Third, change your environment if necessary. If you have been barraged by self-condemning statements and rebuking them hasn't helped, get up and do something. Often just moving to another room will make a difference. Do something to break your thought patterns. Call a friend. Go get a cup of coffee. If you are working on a particularly discouraging project or task, put it aside for the moment and do something different.

Fourth, decide that you are going to embrace the truth about yourself and stop believing the lies. Before you can do this, you will have to know what the truth is. Sometimes it is easier to believe the lies. We can find ourselves agreeing with a subtle lie, "That's right, I'll never really get on top of this weight problem. I've never been able to say no to a chocolate chip cookie." To use the truth effectively, you have got to know what it is.

Here are some examples of lies and self-defeating statements that I have heard from my patients. Perhaps they sound familiar. Along with them, I will put the truth, the positive statement that you should be telling yourself.

1. "I'll never be able to lose this weight. Why bother trying."

You are absolutely right. If you keep thinking like that, you never will. Turn that statement around and start speaking the truth to yourself. You could say something like "Yes, I can and will lose this weight. It's very hard for me, but I have done many hard things, and there's no reason I cannot do this. I need to continue to ask the Lord for strength." You need to make Paul's statement your own: "I can do all things in him who strengthens me" (Col 4:13). Never let anyone, including yourself, tell you that you cannot do it. If you take one step at a time you can.

2. "I went off my diet again. See, I told you I couldn't do it."

Why are we so hard on ourselves when we fail in this area? What happens when you fail in other things? If you become irritable with someone, you probably come back a little later and repent and repair the wrongdoing. But you probably do not berate yourself for the next two days because of it, deciding that you simply are not good enough to be a Christian. You are probably more patient with yourself in other areas of your life than in the area of diet.

When you fail on your diet, in small ways or large, stop worrying about it. Stop hating yourself for it. Just forget it. Put it behind you. It was not the worst thing in the world. It's not necessary to analyze why you went off the diet. Just get right back on track. You may or may not understand eventually why you did it. Turn the lie around. Admit that you made a mistake, but that the world is not coming to an end because of it.

3. "If the Lord loved me, he would help me lose weight."

It's easy to tell yourself this and to keep right on eating whatever you want to. The Lord does love you and will help you, but that does not mean that effort is not required on your part. You must accept the problem and make the best of it. The Lord will give you grace, but you need to ask for it. Sometimes it will be easy, but many times it will not.

4. "I don't deserve to be thin."

Does anyone "deserve" to be thin? Does anyone deserve to be happy? Attractive? Successful? You certainly deserve it as much as anyone else. It may be true that it is easier for some people to stay thin than others, but that doesn't mean that you should not or cannot be thin. It is easier for some people to be good, solid Christians than it is for others, but those who find it difficult should not give up. Think of someone you know who is thin. Does he or she deserve it more than you? Of course not. To say such a thing is almost like saying you do not deserve to have brown hair.

It isn't wrong to want to be thin, healthy, and attractive. Such a desire should not become an idol in your life or occupy an inordinate amount of time and thought, but there is nothing wrong with wanting to lose weight.

When you are actually in the throes of dieting and changing your behavior patterns, your effort can occupy a great deal of time and thought. But controlling your weight will not always require such an investment once things are under control.

If you have made a serious decision to lose weight, get all the tools you can. Read about it; talk about it; pray about it; and think about it. Make it a major part of your life right now. You need all the help you can get. Jump in with both feet. You want to win this game, and you will.

5. "People don't like me because I am fat. If I were thin, they would like me."

For some of us, our extra weight acts as a scapegoat. It can be much less painful to blame our failures on our weight than on ourselves. A common train of thought runs like this, "If I were thin and attractive, I would probably be popular and have lots of dates. One of these days I will decide to lose weight and my life will change. I just haven't decided yet." Such thoughts can be dangerous. Clearly, the extra weight has taken on deeper meaning. What happens if we lose weight? Where would our scapegoat be? What if we didn't have any dates and still felt unpopular? Are we unconsciously afraid to lose the weight and our scapegoat with it?

Very often, scapegoats are ways of dealing with unrealistic expectations. People's opinions of us don't usually depend on whether we are fat or thin. The fact is that some people may never especially like us, regardless of how thin we become. That's life. We need to set realistic goals and expectations for ourselves. We cannot afford to blame failures on our fat.

Are you constantly disappointed with your lot in life because you had expected something better than what you experience now? Accept yourself and your life just the way it is. Embrace it. A scapegoat won't help you deal with it. Of course you can set high goals for yourself, but be sure that they are realistic. If your goal is to become a professional basketball player despite the fact that you are 5'6" and not particularly good at sports, you are bound to become frustrated.

Consider the strengths and gifts that God has given you. Set goals based on these. Ask the Lord to show you what he has for your life. What are his goals for you? If your goals conflict with his, you may, indeed, need a scapegoat on which to blame your failures.

6. "Yes, I am successful at other things, but the fact that I still have a weight problem just shows that I am not *really* a success."

Why do you place so much importance on your weight? Does success or failure seem to hinge on what the scale tells you? Is this God's perspective? Certainly not. Your weight problem is only one aspect of your life. Career is another. Your family is yet another. Each has its place. More important than any of these is your relationship with God. Resist the temptation to make your weight the most important thing in your life.

You may not be doing as well with your weight problem as with some other areas of your life, but that is all right. You will do better eventually. It is a mistake to belittle your success in other areas simply because you still have some work to do in this one.

It's easy in our society to end up with an inferiority complex if you have a weight problem. I have talked with many people of normal weight who consider themselves fat by society's standards. As a result, they constantly struggle to lose weight. Ask the Lord for his perspective on your weight and eating problem. It may be very different from your own. To sum up, take these steps whenever you are having difficulty with lies or negative thoughts.

1. Recognize them for what they are.
2. Stop the thoughts. Rebuke them. Remember, they are not the truth.
3. Change your immediate environment if necessary.
4. Speak the truth to yourself. Yes, you can do it.

Week Twelve Assignment:

Make two columns in your notebook. In the first column list lies that you might hear. List the ones that you can easily deal with, but also list the ones you are convinced of, such as "I will never really lose this weight."

Now, in the second column, write the truth that you are going to tell yourself. State it in a way that is believable to you. For instance, "Losing all this weight seems overwhelming to me, but if I take it one step at a time I can do it. Today I am going to focus on keeping my food diary."

THIRTEEN

It's All Their Fault, or Is It?

THE PEOPLE IN YOUR LIFE can significantly affect your weight problem. A child's social environment holds at least one of the keys as to whether he or she is going to develop a weight problem early in life or later on as an adult. Some children learn early on that Mommy and Daddy are pleased if they eat well. Since they happen to excel in this area, they begin to overeat at the age of two or three, thus developing a serious weight problem as they grow older.

As an adult, the people around you can still affect whether you gain, maintain, or lose weight. It is important to evaluate your current environment and the people in it. How are they affecting you? Can you make changes if necessary?

Some people may send out confusing signals. For instance, you may be famous for your baking skills. You have always received plenty of positive reinforcement for this particular ability. On the other hand, the same people that love and praise you for all the goodies you bake criticize you for your weight problem. They like what you are doing for them, but they abhor what you are doing to yourself. In the midst of such confusing signals, it can be difficult to change your behavior. You enjoy the positive reinforcement but are uncomfortable with criticism. You are trapped in the middle, perhaps without even realizing it.

It is important for you to take charge in a situation like this. Make a decision to diet and to stop baking. Then let people know about it. Some people will be pleased and supportive, but others may not be. A few may actually feel threatened by your decision to lose weight, especially if they could stand to lose a few pounds themselves.

Regardless of how people respond to the news, you need to let them know how they can best support you in your diet. You cannot expect them to read your mind. You are the one who is dieting, and you need to deal with the effects of your diet on others.

Your spouse may surprise you by the way that he or she relates to your decision. Perhaps your wife continues to offer you treats forbidden by your diet. If you refuse, she may feel rebuffed. Communicate directly with her. If you want people to stop rewarding you with sweets or cooking high-calorie meals for you, then you need to let them know that. You can't simply assume that "she knows I am on a diet and can't eat that." Instead, make a specific request for what you want. Most of the time, you will find that people are willing to comply with it. But *you* are the one who must let them know what your needs are.

A patient of mine by the name of Susan had a cousin named Alice who lived near her. Alice knew all of Susan's favorite foods and always provided a special snack whenever Susan came to visit. Alice knew that Susan was serious about her diet, but she continued to provide special treats every time Susan visited. Finally, Susan got up the courage to tell Alice that she appreciated the treats but could not eat them because of her new diet. She then gave her cousin some ideas about how to express her love and support for her, like providing iced tea, diet pop, low-calorie ice milk, or some other kind of treat that she could have. Alice complied eagerly and offered her the right kinds of food whenever she visited. She even went a step beyond Susan's advice and kept cookies and other treats out of sight. This helped Susan tremendously. From then on, she never hesitated to tell people exactly what she wanted or needed, though she was careful not to do it in a critical way.

Should I Ask for Compliments?

The answer is yes. It is worth asking for compliments. A compliment that you have asked for is just as valuable as a compliment that is freely given. Very often, your friends and relatives do not know quite what to say to encourage you. As a result, they may say nothing. They may feel awkward telling you how well you are doing on your diet, how good you look, or how well you handled that party. If you ask for input, you will usually find that people will give it gladly.

You might say something like this to your husband as you leave a party: "Didn't I handle that party well?" Your comment gives him an opening to compliment you by saying something like, "You really did. I noticed that you refused to eat even one of the hors d'oeuvres." If you don't occasionally open the door for such compliments, people may feel that your diet is none of their business.

So if you feel in need of a compliment, ask for one, from a friend, a relative, or someone else that you can trust.

Social Pressure to Eat: How Can I Resist?

Never let yourself eat because you think it is the "courteous" thing to do, or because you are pressured to eat. If you had a medical problem like diabetes or hypertension, you wouldn't let people pressure you to eat things that would make the problem worse.

When you say, "No, thank you," make it firm, straightforward, and direct. If you sound uncertain, you will only invite more pressure. Say, "No, thank you. I'm not eating desserts right now." A response like "Well, I really shouldn't but . . ." only invites the host or hostess to twist your arm gently, persuading you to eat the very thing that you should avoid at all costs.

Recently, I attended a dinner party with a prominent local physician. I was impressed to notice that he refused to let himself be pressured to eat dessert. The dinner and the desserts were made by some lovely women. After dinner, five different desserts were offered. Many of the guests were sampling a small piece of each of the desserts. The women were delighted with everyone's enthusiasm. When this particular doctor was asked what he would like, he responded politely, but firmly, saying, "No, thank you. I never eat desserts." And that was that. Because he said it so firmly and directly they were not tempted to pressure him to "have just a little piece."

More often than not, people care less about what we eat than we think they do. Marilyn, another of my patients, had been invited out for ice cream. She and her date were going with another couple to a nearby ice-cream parlor. She decided ahead of time to order iced tea rather than ice cream. But in the days preceding the date she was anxious and upset, certain that the other people in her little group would pressure her to eat ice cream.

Finally, the moment came. Her date didn't bat an eye when she ordered iced tea. He ordered a cup of coffee for himself. The other couple had ice cream, and no one said a thing about it. Clearly, they couldn't have cared less what Marilyn ordered.

Many of us are afraid that we will hurt someone's feelings if we refuse their food. But nine times out of ten, people really don't care that much. So never let people pressure you into eating things that you have decided not to eat.

Sabotage and How to Deal with It

Has anyone tried to sabotage your diet? Have you noticed that a friend consistently offers you high-calorie food even after you have asked him not to? There are reasons for such sabotage.

Perhaps that person envies your success. He may prefer you the way you were. Quite commonly, your former eating partner is the culprit. This person could be your spouse or a close friend, with whom you used to overeat. You went to the theater and ate treats from the snack bar. You ordered to the ice-cream shop together. Now that you are on a diet, you still want to spend time with him, but you are not willing to eat with him anymore. Without meaning to, you may be making this person feel guilty. If you drink a cup of coffee while he eats a sundae, he will probably feel uncomfortable and guilty. Would you please eat a hot fudge sundae with him? To resist this kind of pressure, you will need to deal with your own discomfort and your friend's attempt at sabotage.

It helps to recognize that this person is having a difficult time with the fact that you are dieting. It may be possible to discuss it with him. Or it may be wiser to let him handle his own feelings about the situation. He may not even be very aware that he is trying to sabotage your diet. In time, he will be able to accept the change in you, and his efforts at sabotage will diminish and probably disappear.

Announce Your Intentions

Announcing your intentions can prove to be a helpful technique in social situations. It can enable you to maintain your resolve to stick to your diet. You make your intention "public" by telling at least one other person or perhaps a whole group that you are not going to eat something in a particular situation. By doing this, you are burning your bridges behind you, cutting off all the options. Having told others of your intention, you are not likely to give in to temptation.

Suppose you are at the office, and you receive a five-pound box of chocolates from one of your clients. They happen to be your favorite kind. You could say to yourself, "I am not going to eat any of those. In fact, I am not even going to go into the lounge where they are." But you say nothing to anyone. You could change your mind. After all, who would know? An hour or two later you could relent and say, "Maybe I will just have one."

A wiser approach would be to tell at least one other person about your decision. Say, "Don't let me eat any of those chocolates. In fact, please keep them out of my sight." Such a statement makes it very difficult for you to change your mind.

This technique works for me frequently, especially when my husband and I are going to a party. Before the party, I might say something like, "I am not going to eat anything tonight. If you see me eating, you have my permission to come up and nudge me." He never says anything out loud or does anything to embarrass me. But if I have asked him to keep his eye on me, I know that I will stick to my decision.

Whenever you announce your intention, be sure that you mean what you say. It does no good, and even some harm, to make a statement that you are likely to contradict minutes later. If you do, people will not take you seriously in the future.

Humor Can Make the Difference

Losing weight need not be an intense and humorless undertaking. Your efforts to diet and to apply the behavior-change techniques we have discussed will be greatly enhanced if you approach them with a sense of humor. For instance, if someone does bring a box of chocolates into your office and offers you one, don't jump to the conclusion that they are trying to sabotage your diet. Joke about it or say something teasingly about it. But use your sense of humor to enlist support from others. It doesn't help to be tense and defensive about what you are doing. Relax. Joke about your inability to cope with a piece of chocolate cake. If you make light of it in a good-natured and not in a negative way, you will receive a lot more cooperation and understanding from those around you.

"I Will Only Love You If You Are Thin"

Have you ever felt that some people base their love for you on whether you are fat or thin? Perhaps your mother constantly rem   "Sally, can't you lose that weight? You would be so   er." She may think that she is loving you by being   ut your weight, but her words make it clear that   ting up to her expectations.

sibility to let people know how such attitudes

affect you. Tell them that you need their love and support, but that you need it unconditionally. It makes life difficult for you if they only approve of you when you are thin. You need their consistent love and concern to help give you the strength and motivation to remain on your diet.

Jane, a patient of mine, lost a good deal of weight. Several of her husband's friends asked him what he had done to help her lose so much weight. "Nothing," he said. "I loved her and supported her like I always do, but I let her handle her weight problem herself. I complimented her if she wanted compliments. But basically, I just let her know that I loved her." He told them that he had reached a point in their relationship when he realized that he loved her regardless of whether she lost the weight. His love had nothing to do with what size clothes she wore. The knowledge of his love gave her tremendous freedom to try something new. She could attempt to lose the weight with the assurance that she would not be letting him down if she failed. She succeeded, and they were both pleased. Even so, her husband's pleasure at her weight loss did not affect his love or concern for her. He had already accepted her as she was.

Weight-Control Groups

No one statement applies to every weight-control group. They vary tremendously from place to place and from one type of group to another. The strength of any one group depends to a great extent on the person who leads it. If you are considering joining a weight-control program or group, go to a meeting and observe the leader. Talk to him or her. Make your decision on the basis of whether he or she is someone you can respect and trust.

It is helpful to look to someone else for guidance about your diet. You will want to choose someone you trust and respect— your doctor, dietician, nurse, or the leader of a weight-control group. You should be able to talk over your difficulties with them, to receive advice and encouragement.

Some groups can provide help for you even if the leader is not a person who inspires great respect. The teaching they offer can be valuable in itself. If they use a behavior-modification program, you may be able to go to the group meetings for information that you can use on your own.

Whenever you are in a weight-control group, listen discerningly. It is unwise to believe and absorb everything you hear. Don't let the philosophy of the leader or the group form or mold you. Take from the situation whatever will help you lose weight, and leave behind the things that you disagree with. Many weight-control groups reflect a secular worldview and a self-centered philosophy. Discard whatever is contrary to your Christian life and your desire to follow the Lord.

It may not be possible to find the ideal type of support, but refuse to let this fact be an excuse for not losing weight. It can be easy to blame your weight problem on your dislike of groups or of diet food. Take whatever help you can find and make the best of it. If you wanted to learn how to type, you would take a typing class. The same is true of losing weight. You need to learn how to do it. You can't simply assume that you know how.

It is usually best to join a weight-control group that costs money rather than one that is free. Paying for something means that you are serious about it, that you are committed to it. This is not to say that a group that costs you nothing will not be of help, but only that it may elicit less commitment from you.

It can be embarrassing to go to a weight-control group. After all, you may not want to associate with "fat" people. You may hope that no one will see you walk in the door. But it is freeing to take that step and to say to yourself, "I admit my weight problem. These people are also overweight. They are working to do something about it and I can too."

By refusing to get help, you deny your problem and say to yourself that you are different from those other people. Your weight problem is different than theirs. You can lose weight once you decide to. You just haven't decided yet.

This kind of an attitude can prevent you from receiving the very help that can make a difference for you. So put aside your pride and look for a weight-control group. Or go to your doctor or to a weight therapist where you can get some help and some teaching. Never be embarrassed about needing help. If you could handle it on your own, you wouldn't have a weight problem in the first place.

Week Thirteen Assignment:

1. Make a list of all the people in your life who are very supportive of your diet. Make a second list of people who are not so supportive. Next to the names in the second list, write your plan. Decide how you will talk to each one or what you can do to elicit their support. Remember, they can't read your mind. Ask for the kind of support you need.
2. Write down social situations where you find it difficult to diet. Draw up a plan for dealing with each one.

FOURTEEN

Maintaining
Your Weight Loss

YOU HAVE BEEN DIETING and working on your eating behavior for several weeks now, and you have lost seventeen pounds. But you still have fifteen to go. To tell the truth, you are getting tired of it. It is not quite as easy as it was at first, and your motivation seems to be slipping away. After all, you can fit into that navy blue suit that had gotten too tight. And you are getting lots of compliments about how good you look. You are wondering whether you really need or want to go on.

It is at just such times that you may find yourself eating more than you should. Once this happens, the guilt, self-condemnation, and hopelessness begin. Don't give in to them. If you eat a high-calorie treat forget it. Pick yourself up and keep right on going. If you stop to let the guilt and self-condemnation surge in and take over, you are only going to have a bigger battle to fight. It rarely helps to spend a lot of time trying to figure out why you ate something you shouldn't have. Make sure that the very next thing you eat *is* on your diet. Even if you ate shortly before dinner, don't skip dinner as a way to make up for the mistake. If you do, you will be hungry about nine or ten o'clock and will feel deprived because you skipped dinner. Chances are you will go off your diet again.

Helps and Hindrances

Take out a piece of paper. Make two columns. Label one "Helps" and the other "Hindrances." In the "Helps" column, list everything you can think of that helps you stay on your diet. In the "Hindrances" column, list anything that makes it more difficult for you. List all your stumbling blocks, whether they be certain kinds of food, certain places, or certain people.

Helps	*Hindrances*
a regular schedule	being out of town
enough sleep	business luncheons
fruit	baking
big salads	the bakery
being at work	the pizza restaurant
visiting the Smith's	visiting my cousin, Susie

You may have fifteen or twenty items in each column, or more. You want to be clear about which things are helpful for you and which are stumbling blocks. Focus on the helps. It is much easier to start doing something than to stop doing something. Concentrate your efforts on doing the things that help rather than expending all your energy avoiding the things that are difficulties. "Lean into" the helps and "lean away" from the hindrances.

Keep your list handy so that you will see it and it will stay fresh in your mind. If you can avoid the hindrances, then do. If you can just as easily schedule a business meeting for 10:00 in the morning over coffee, rather than at noon over lunch, then do that. If you can choose another route to work rather than one that passes by the front door of the bakery, then do that. If you find that you have to do something in the "hindrance" column, then plan it carefully. If you have your defenses ready and use them, you will be safe.

Holidays and Vacations

You may find that you still gain weight on holidays or whenever you take a vacation. The most important thing is to return to your normal way of eating as soon as the holiday or vacation is over. Regardless of whether they are overweight or thin, most people gain during holidays and while on vacations. The difference is that thin people make a point of losing the extra weight right away so it has no chance to accumulate month after month and year after year. If you let yourself gain five pounds every Christmas, and make no effort to lose it, that will add up to fifty pounds in ten years!

Another commonsense principle to resort to on holidays is to get rid of the leftovers. If your feast on Thanksgiving extends for three days rather than one, you are in trouble. But if you prepare only enough food to last for the meal itself, you will be much better off.

Maintenance

When you set a goal weight, give yourself a five-pound range. For instance, if your goal is 135 pounds, your range would be 133-138. Since your weight fluctuates naturally from day to day, you should expect that on some days you will weigh less and on some days more. If you surpass the top of your range, go back to the original diet. As long as you are within your range, you can follow a maintenance plan.

Maintenance is quite simple and even fun. Once you reach your goal weight, you can begin. Here is how it works.

Maintenance, Week One—You may add 100 calories a day, or 700 a week, to the regular diet that you have been following. You may use them however you like. Some of my patients like to use the extra calories by adding something each day, say an extra ounce of cheese or an extra ounce of cereal. Many people like to stay on their regular diet Monday through Friday and then use their extra calories on the weekend. If you do that, then this week you have 700 calories to use. You could use it for dessert on Saturday night and coffee cake on Sunday morning. Think about how you would like to use the extra calories and then make your plan.

Maintenance, Week Two—At the end of the week, weigh

yourself. If you are still within your goal range, give yourself another 100 calories per day. Now you have 200 extra calories a day, or 1,400 extra for the week. Again, you may use them however you like. You may use them all on the weekend or spread them throughout the week.

Maintenance, Week Three—At the end of week two, weigh yourself. If you are still within your goal range, you may give yourself an additional 100 calories per day, or a total of 2,100 extra for the week.

Simply continue this way until you start to gain. When you do, you know that you have hit your limit. You may find that your maintenance level is the basic diet plus 300 calories per day. Each person is a little different. It will depend on whether you are a man or a woman, whether you are physically active, and whether your calorie estimates are accurate.

If you do not have a good calorie-counter book, you will need one. *Calories and Carbohydrates,* by Barbara Kraus, has the advantage of being both comprehensive and inexpensive.

When you begin maintenance, continue to use all the techniques you have learned. Keep your food diary during this time and sit at your designated eating place. Eat slowly and resist buying high-calorie impulse foods.

If you want to eat ice cream to use up your extra calories this week, go ahead. But never buy a half gallon to bring home. Go out to a restaurant or ice-cream parlor and eat it there. You will not be faced with half a carton of ice cream in your freezer the next day.

One of my patients had reached her goal weight and was on maintenance. She decided to buy a coffee cake for Sunday breakfast. She thought she could handle it and decided to try. But the leftovers got the best of her. Having all that coffee cake in the house was just a little more than she could handle. But she learned something from the experience. From then on she avoided coffee cake and bought other treats for Sunday morning, ones that didn't tempt her so much.

Once you start maintenance, don't become discouraged by little mistakes. The techniques we have discussed are designed not only to help you lose weight but to help you keep it off. This is a time of experimenting and testing what you can handle and what you cannot. You are going to be eating things you haven't eaten in a long while, and you shouldn't expect perfection. Remember, you are learning.

Week Fourteen Assignment:

1. The following check list (fig. 11) is designed to help you with your maintenance plan. Some of the behaviors that you should continue working on are listed. Fill in the blank spaces with the particular behaviors you think you should be working on, perhaps keeping track of your sleep or exercise.

2. Use the Maintenance Calorie Counter (fig. 12) to keep track of how many extra calories you use per day. The example for Week 1 of the chart shows that you can use 700 calories more than your regular diet during that week. For each day of the week, the number left of the slash mark shows the calories consumed that day. The number to the right of the mark shows the running total for the week. In the example, no extra calories were used on Monday. On Tuesday, 100 were used. 150 of the extra calories were used on Wednesday, so the running total for the week is 250. Thus the Wednesday entry is marked 150/250. The days during the rest of the week are marked accordingly, with the total allowance of 700 calories having been used by Sunday.

The second week shows that you have 1400 extra calories to use however you like. Record your use of them in the same way that you did for Week 1.

Add 700 calories each successive week as long as you are within your desired weight range.

Figure 11
Daily Checklist for Week of _____

Behavior	M	T	W	Th	F	Sat	S
Kept Food Diary							
Designated Eating Place							
Stayed on Diet Consistently							

Date _____ **Weight** _____

Sample
Daily Checklist for Week of ___ _8/17_ ___

Behavior	M	T	W	Th	F	Sat	S
Kept Food Diary	✓		✓	✓	✓	✓	✓
Designated Eating Place	✓	✓	✓	✓	✓	✓	✓
Stayed on Diet Consistently	✓	✓	✓	✓		✓	✓
Exercise	ran 20 min.		ran 20 min		ran 20 min		
Got enough sleep	7 hrs.	7 hrs.	8½ hrs	8 hrs	6½ hrs	7½ hrs	8 hrs.

Date _8/20_ **Weight** _160_

Figure 12

Maintenance Calorie Counter

Extra Calories Per Week	Monday	Tuesday	Wednesday	Thursday	Friday	Saturday	Sunday
Week 1 700 Cal	0/0	100/100	150/250	0/250	250/500	0/600	200/700
Week 2 1400 Cal							
Week 3							
Week 4							
Week 5							
Week 6							
Week 7							
Week 8							

FIFTEEN

The Long Run

I F YOU HAVE BEEN thin before, you know that all the trouble it takes to get there is worth it. If you have never been thin, let me assure you that it is well worth the struggle, the stress, and even the tears. It is worth it not just because you will look and feel better but because you will know that at long last you are in charge of your desires for food. They are no longer in charge of you. You know that you can say yes when you want to and no when you want to. Food no longer runs the show. You do.

Because eating is a self-reinforcing behavior, it is a very difficult though not impossible one to change. Few personal problems are as difficult to change as a weight problem, but few can teach you so many helpful things about life. Very often, the determining factor will be your persistence. Working at it, day in and day out, week in and week out can build character. It can strengthen you. As Paul says in his letter to the Romans:

> We rejoice in our sufferings, knowing that suffering produces endurance, and endurance produces character, and character produces hope, and hope does not disappoint us, because God's love has been poured into our hearts through the Holy Spirit which has been given to us. (Rom 5:3)

The fruit of your efforts is not just a thinner body, but a stronger spirit. You *can* control your impulses. You can be in charge.

Losing weight bears many similarities to the rest of your Christian life. You know that life is a struggle that will not be over until you are at last with the Lord. You don't let yourself become discouraged and quit. You don't say to yourself, "If I can't be a perfect Christian in three months, then it isn't worth it, and I am not even going to try." You expect life to be an ongoing struggle, one in which you will experience victories and defeats. But you push on, assured that, ultimately, the victory will be yours.

Try to view your weight problem in the same way. Losing weight is going to be an ongoing process. You will never be able to go back to the old habits if you want to stay in control.

Thank God for your weight problem. Does that sound ridiculous? It isn't. Your weight problem can be an opportunity for God to work in your life. If nothing else keeps you on your knees before the Lord, it will. Keep admitting your weakness to him. As you do, he will give you the strength and grace to deal with it. He may not take away the problem in an instant, but he will give you what you need to meet it head on and win.

God can give you the tools, but you need to pick them up and use them. Through your persistence the Lord will work. He will use this very weakness to build you up that you may give glory to him. Paul says, "A thorn was given me in the flesh . . . to harass me, to keep me from being too elated. Three times I besought the Lord about this, that it should leave me; but he said to me, 'My grace is sufficient for you, for my power is made perfect in weakness'" (2 Cor 12:7-9).

Gaining Confidence

Your confidence in this area will spill over into other areas. Feeling weak and helpless in the face of food affects the way you feel about yourself in the face of more intimidating obstacles. But if you begin to experience one victory after another in your struggles with food, you will have more confidence and self-esteem to handle other areas of your life.

There is something to say for being more attractive, too. It is true that people are generally more attracted to people who look fit. Being thin and more attractive is not a bad thing to desire. If you feel good about the way you look, you will act more confidently in all you do, whether it involves giving a presentation at work or a teaching from the pulpit. Your appearance is certainly not the most important thing in life, but it is a significant part of who you are. If you can enhance it without falling into vanity, go ahead.

If you lose weight, you are sure to feel better physically. You will not tire as easily, and you will find it easier to move around. You won't be huffing and puffing after walking half a block. Losing weight will take extra strain off your joints and back as well as your heart, lungs, and other organs. You will probably live a longer and healthier life.

Your efforts at losing weight can greatly encourage others. As they see your perseverance pay off, they may begin to think, "If he could do it, maybe I can." Your success can be the glimmer of hope they need. Never flaunt your success or criticize others for their seeming lack of motivation. Remember, you were once in their position. Your good example can be the first step to their own eventual victory.

God's Perspective

If you think that losing weight and being thin is the most important thing in life, you are wrong. That is not God's perspective. Many things are more important—your relationship with the Lord, your relationships with others, the responsibilities God has given you, to name just a few.

If losing weight holds too much meaning and importance for you, it is only going to make the battle harder. Every time you experience a little failure, it will seem monumental. You will hate yourself for being overweight and project that self-hatred to those around you.

What is your most hideous and deplorable weakness? Is it your weight problem? In the midst of great weakness, God can manifest great strength. Let him do that for you. You can beg him to take away your weight problem, and he may do that. But he will probably use it to purify you—to strengthen and build your character. You may succeed in every area of your life but this one. Thank God for your weakness if it brings you back to the Lord again and again on your knees, asking for his help and his grace.

The Lord God loves you right now, just the way you are. He is not withholding his love until you reach your goal weight. You need to love and accept yourself now, just as you are. If thinness has become an idol in your life, let go of it and ask God for his perspective. He will give it to you.

Notes

1. A.J. Stunkard, Presidential Address—1974: "From Explanation to Action in Psychosomatic Medicine: The Case of Obesity," *Psychosomatic Medicine,* vol. 37, no. 3 (May-June 1975), pp. 199-203.

2. "One-Hundred Leading National Advertisers," *Advertising Age* (September 9, 1982), p. 8.

3. T.W. Leed and G.A. German, *Food Merchandising: Principles and Practices* (New York: Chain Store Publishing Corp., Subsidiary of Lebhar-Friedman, Inc., 1979), p. 270.

4. *Ibid.,* p. 293.

5. *Ibid.,* p. 347.

6. *The Colonial Study* (New York: Progressive Grocer, 1963), pp. 126-27.

7. A.J. Stunkard, *I Almost Feel Thin* (Palo Alto, California: Bull Publishing Co., 1977), p. 74.

Bibliography

Cooper, K., *The New Aerobics* (New York: Bantam, 1970).

Cooper, M., and Cooper, K., *Aerobics for Women* (New York: Bantam, 1970).

Cross, J., *The Supermarket Trap* (Bloomington: Indiana University Press, 1970).

Dobson, James, *Hide or Seek* (Old Tappan, New Jersey: Revell, 1974).

Eat and Stay Slim (Des Moines, Iowa: Meredith Corp., Better Homes and Gardens, Consumer Book Div., 1980).

Edelstein, Barbara, *The Woman Doctor's Diet for Women* (New York: Ballantine Books, 1977).

Fanburg, W.H., and Snyder, B.S., *How to be a Winner at the Weight Loss Game* (New York: Ballantine, 1975).

Ferguson, J.M., *Habit, Not Diets* (Palo Alto, California: Bull Publishing, 1976).

Ferguson, J.M., *Learning to Eat: Behavior Modification for Weight Control* (Palo Alto, California: Bull Publishing, 1975).

Ikeda, J., *For Teenagers Only: Change Your Habits to Change Your Shape* (Palo Alto, California: Bull Publishing, 1978).

Jeffrey, D., and Katz, R., *Take It Off and Keep It Off: A Behavioral Program for Weight Loss and Healthful Living* (Englewood Cliffs, New Jersey: Prentice-Hall, 1977).

Jordan, H.A., Levitz, L.S., and Kimbrell, G.M., *Eating Is Okay* (New York: Signet, 1976).

Kraus, Barbara, *Calories and Carbohydrates* (New York: Signet, 1981).

Kress, G., *Marketing Research* (Reston, Virginia: Reston Publishing Company, Inc., 1979).

LaHaye, Tim, *How to Win Over Depression* (Grand Rapids, Michigan: Zondervan, 1974).

Leed, T.W., and German, G.A., *Food Merchandising: Principles and Practices* (New York: Chain Store Publishing Corp., A Subsidiary of Lebhar-Friedman, Inc., 1979).

Lewis, H.G., *How to Make Your Advertising Twice as Effective at Half the Cost* (Chicago: Nelson-Hall, 1979).

Maas, J., *Better Brochures, Catalogs and Mailing Pieces* (New York: St. Martin's Press, 1981).

Marion, B.W., Mueller, W.F., Cotterill, R.W., Geithman, F.E., Schmelzer, J.R., *The Food Retailing Industry: Market Structure, Profits, and Prices* (New York: Praeger Publishers, Praeger Special Studies, 1979).

151

Marquette, A.F., *Brands, Trademarks and Good Will* (New York: McGraw-Hill, 1967).

Nash, J.D., and Long, L.O., *Taking Charge of Your Weight and Well-Being* (Palo Alto, California: Bull Publishing, 1978).

Ogilvy, D., *Confessions of an Advertising Man* (New York: Atheneum, 1981, first printing, 1963).

Orbach, S., *Fat Is a Feminist Issue* (New York: Berkley Publications, 1979).

Pleuthner, W.A., *460 Secrets of Advertising Experts* (Nashville, Tennessee: Thomas Nelson & Sons, 1961).

Redd, W.H., Porterfield, A.L., and Andersen, B.L., *Behavior Modification: Behavioral Approaches to Human Problems* (New York: Random House, 1979).

Reeves, R., *Reality in Advertising* (New York: Alfred A. Knopf, 1977).

Roman, K., and Maas, J., *How to Advertise* (New York: St. Martin's Press, 1976).

Rubin, T.I., *Alive and Fat and Thinning in America* (New York: Coward, McCann and Geoghegan, Inc., 1978).

Rubin, Theodore S., *Forever Thin* (New York: Berkley Publications, 1970).

Schaeffer, Edith: *Hidden Art* (Wheaton, Illinois: Tyndale Publishers, 1971).

Seiden, Hank, *Advertising Pure and Simple* (New York, AMACOM, 1976).

Shedd, Charles, *The Fat Is in Your Head* (Waco, Texas: Word Books, 1972).

Stuart, R.B., *Act Thin, Stay Thin* (New York: W.W. Norton and Co., 1978).

Stuart, R.B., and Davis, B., *Slim Chance in a Fat World* (Champaign, Illinois: Research Press, 1972).

Stunkard, A.J., Presidential Address—1974: "From Explanation to Action in Psychosomatic Medicine: the Case of Obesity," *Psychosomatic Medicine,* vol. 37, no. 3 (May-June 1975): 195-236.

Stunkard, A.J., *I Almost Feel Thin* (Palo Alto, California: Bull Publishing, 1977).

Watson, D.L., and Tharp, R.J., *Self-Directed Behavior,* second edition (Monterey, California: Brooks/Cole Publishing Co., 1977).

1974 Food Shopping Habits Study of Super Market Shoppers: Their Buying Habits and Attitudes (Cincinnati, Ohio: Burgoyne, Inc.: October, 1974).

Suggested Reading

Behavior Change

Ferguson, J.M., *Habit, Not Diets* (Palo Alto, California: Bull Publishing, 1976).
A useful do-it-yourself behavior change program.

Jeffrey, D., and Ratz, R., *Take It Off and Keep It Off: A Behavioral Program for Weight Loss and Healthful Living* (Englewood Cliffs, New Jersey: Prentice-Hall, 1977).

Jordan, H.A., Levitz, L.S., and Kimbrell, G.M., *Eating Is Okay* (New York: Signet, 1976).

Nash, J.D., and Long, L.O., *Taking Charge of Your Weight and Well-Being* (Palo Alto, California: Bull Publishing, 1978).
Complete but very lengthy.

Stuart, R.B., and Davis, B., *Slim Chance in a Fat World* (Champaign, Illinois: Research Press Co., 1972).
Excellent but technical.

Watson, D.L., and Tharp, R.G., *Self-Directed Behavior,* second edition (Monterey, California: Brooks/Cole Publishing Co., 1977).
Excellent textbook for teaching how to develop behavior change programs for altering undesirable behaviors or beginning new behaviors.

Exercise

Cooper, K., *The New Aerobics* (New York: Bantam, 1970).
Cooper, M., and Cooper, K., *Aerobics for Women* (New York: Bantam, 1970).

Nutrition

Eat and Stay Slim (Des Moines, Iowa: Meredith Corp., Better Homes and Gardens, Consumer Book Div., 1980).

Kraus, Barbara, *Calories and Carbohydrates* (New York: Signet, 1981).

Gibbons, Barbara, *Diet Watchers Cookbook* (Skokie, Illinois: Consumer Guide, Nov. 1977, vol. 161).

Diabetic Cookbook
Recipes are based on the exchange type diet and can easily be used in conjunction with the diet on the *Winning at Losing* plan. The book is available from the Department of Food and Nutrition Services, St. John's Hospital, 300 E. Carpenter, Springfield, Illinois 62702.

Additional Reading

Dobson, James, *Hide or Seek* (Old Tappan, New Jersey: Revell, 1974).
Excellent suggestions for children, teenagers, or adults on coping with "handicaps" such as being overweight. Gives perspective on how to develop healthy self-esteem regardless of what difficulties may face an individual.

Felton, Sandra, *The Messies' Manual.*
Helpful guide to housekeeping for women. Having order in one area of your life carries over to other areas. Can be obtained from Writer's Service, P.O. Box 152, Miami Springs, Florida 33166.

Ghezzi, Bert, *The Angry Christian* (Ann Arbor, Michigan: Servant Books, 1980).

Jackson, Carole, *Color Me Beautiful* (New York: Ballantine, 1981).
Useful guide to choosing color in dress and makeup for women. Exercise caution in reading this. She seems to promise that the right colors will solve all your problems.

LaHaye, Tim, *How to Win Over Depression* (Grand Rapids, Michigan: Zondervan, 1974).
Helpful wisdom on depression and self-pity.

Lakein, A., *How to Get Control of Your Time and Life* (New York: New American Library, 1974).
Helpful, concise guide to identifying priorities in your life and managing your time wisely.

Molloy, J.T., *Dress for Success* (New York: Warner, 1975).
A guide to dress for men. Simple and helpful. Of course, very secular approach but some useful principles.

Molloy, J.T., *The Women's Dress for Success Book* (New York: Warner, 1978).
Women's version of the above.

Rubin, Theodore S., *Forever Thin* (New York: Berkley Publishing Corp., 1970).
Some good insights into weight problems from a psychological perspective.

Schaeffer, Edith, *Hidden Art* (Wheaton, Illinois: Tyndale Publishers, 1971).
Aimed at women. Creative ideas for better use of time, energies, and gifts.

Shedd, Charles, *The Fat Is in Your Head* (Waco, Texas: Word Books, 1972).
A psychological approach with a Christian perspective. I always recommend this book to my patients.

Stunkard, A.J., *I Almost Feel Thin* (Palo Alto, California: Bull Publishing, 1977).
Case histories of patients with severe eating disorders. Discusses treatment with behavior modification. Also published as *The Pain of Obesity.*

Food and Behavior Diary Pages for One Week

Food Diary Page for Monday

Date _____

Time	Place	Activity	Feeling	With Whom	Hunger	Food

Food Diary Page for Tuesday

Date _____

Time	Place	Activity	Feeling	With Whom	Hunger	Food

Food Diary Page for Wednesday

Date_____

Time	Place	Activity	Feeling	With Whom	Hunger	Food

Food Diary Page for Thursday

Date _____

Time	Place	Activity	Feeling	With Whom	Hunger	Food

Food Diary Page for Friday

Date _____

Time	Place	Activity	Feeling	With Whom	Hunger	Food

Food Diary Page for Saturday

Date _____

Time	Place	Activity	Feeling	With Whom	Hunger	Food

Food Diary Page for Sunday

Date _____

Time	Place	Activity	Feeling	With Whom	Hunger	Food

Calorie Equivalents

Dairy Products	*Calories*
Cheese:	
Natural:	
Blue, 1 oz.	100
Cheddar, 1 oz.	115
Cottage, creamed, 1 cup	235
Cream, 1 oz.	100
Mozzarella, 1 oz.	90
Parmesan, grated, 1 tbsp. 25	
Swiss, 1 oz.	105
Pasteurized process cheese	95
food, American, 1 oz.	
Cream, sweet:	
Half-and-half, 1 tbsp.	20
Whipping, heavy, unwhipped:	
1 cup	820
1 tbsp.	80
Cream, sour:	
1 cup	495
1 tbsp.	25
Cream products, sweet:	
Creamers:	
Liquid (frozen), 1 tbsp.	20
Powdered, 1 tsp.	10
Whipped topping, frozen:	
1 cup	240
1 tbsp.	15

Milk:

Whole (3.3% fat), 1 cup	150
Lowfat (2%), 1 cup	120
Lowfat (1%), 1 cup	100
Nonfat (skim), 1 cup	85
Buttermilk, 1 cup	100
Evaporated, unsweetened, canned:	
Whole, 1 cup	340
Skim, 1 cup	200
Dried, nonfat instant, 1 cup powder	245

Milk desserts, frozen:

Ice cream:

Regular (about 11% fat), hardened, 1 cup	270
Rich (about 16% fat), hardened, 1 cup	350
Ice Milk (about 4.3% fat), hardened, 1 cup	185

Yogurt:

Made with lowfat milk:

Fruit-flavored, 8 oz.	230
Plain, 8 oz.	145
Made with nonfat milk, 8 oz.	125

Eggs

Eggs, large:

Whole, 1	80
White, 1	15
Yolk, 1	65

Fats, Oils

Butter:

1 stick (½ cup)	815
1 tbsp.	100
Fats, cooking (vegetable shortenings):	
1 cup	1,770
1 tbsp.	110
Lard:	
1 cup	1,850
1 tbsp.	115

Margarine:

Regular:

1 stick (½ cup)	815
1 tbsp.	100
Soft (2 8-oz. containers per lb.), 1 container	1,635

Oils, salad or cooking:

Corn, 1 tbsp.	120
Olive, 1 tbsp.	120
Peanut, 1 tbsp.	120

Salad dressings, commercial:

Blue Cheese:

Regular, 1 tbsp.	75
Low-calorie (5 cal. per tsp.), 1 tbsp.	15

French:

Regular, 1 tbsp.	65
Low-calorie (5 cal. per tsp.), 1 tbsp.	15

Italian:

Regular, 1 tbsp.	85
Low-calorie (2 cal. per tsp.), 1 tbsp.	10
Mayonnaise, 1 tbsp.	100
Tartar sauce, 1 tbsp.	75

Thousand Island:

Regular, 1 tbsp.	80
Low-calorie (10 cal. per tsp.), 1 tbsp.	25

Fish, Shellfish, Meat, Poultry, Related Products

Fish and shellfish:

Clams:

Fresh, meat only, 3 oz.	65
Canned, solids and liquid, 3 oz.	45
Crabmeat (white or king), canned, 1 cup	135
Fish sticks, breaded, cooked, frozen, 1 stick or 1 oz.	50
Oysters, fresh, meat only (13-19 medium selects), 1 cup	160
Salmon, pink, canned, solids and liquid, 3 oz.	120
Sardines, Atlantic, canned in oil, drained solids, 3 oz.	175
Shrimp, canned, meat only, 3 oz.	100

Tuna, canned in oil, drained solids, 3 oz.	170
Meat and meat products:	
Bacon, broiled or fried, crisp, 2 slices	85
Beef, cooked:	
Lean and fat, 3 oz.	245
Ground beef, broiled:	
Lean with 10% fat, 3 oz.	185
Lean with 21% fat, 2.9 oz.	235
Roast, oven-cooked:	
Relatively fat, such as rib:	
Lean and fat, 3 oz.	375
Lean only, 1.8 oz.	125
Relatively lean, such as heel of round:	
Lean and fat, 3 oz.	165
Steak:	
Relatively fat sirloin, broiled:	
Lean and fat, 3 oz.	330
Lean only, 2 oz.	115
Relatively lean round, braised:	
Lean and fat, 3 oz.	220
Beef, corned, 3 oz.	185
Beef, dried, chipped, 2½-oz. jar	145
Heart, beef, lean, braised, 3 oz.	160
Lamb, cooked:	
Chop, rib:	
Lean and fat, 3.1 oz.	360
Lean only, 2 oz.	120
Leg, roasted:	
Lean and fat, 3 oz.	235
Lean only, 2.5 oz.	130
Shoulder, roasted:	
Lean and fat, 3 oz.	285
Lean only, 2.3 oz.	130
Liver, beef, fried, 3 oz.	195
Pork, cured, cooked:	
Ham, light cure, lean and fat, roasted, 3 oz.	245
Luncheon ham (boiled), 1 oz. slice	65
Pork, fresh, cooked:	
Chop, loin:	
Lean and fat, 2.7 oz.	305

Roast, oven-cooked, no liquid added:
  Lean and fat, 3 oz.   310
Shoulder cut, simmered:
  Lean and fat, 3 oz.   320
Sausages:
  Bologna, 1 oz.   85
  Braunschweiger, 1 oz.   90
  Brown and serve, browned, 1 link   70
  Deviled ham, canned, 1 tbsp.   45
  Frankfurter (8 per 1-lb. pkg.), 1   170
  Vienna sausage, 1   40
Veal, medium fat, cooked, deboned:
  Cutlet, 3 oz.   185
  Rib, 3 oz.   230

Poultry and poultry products:
  Chicken, cooked:
    Breast (½), fried, deboned, 2.8 oz.   160
    Drumstick (1), fried, deboned, 1.3 oz 90
    Half broiler, broiled, deboned, 6.2 oz. 240
  Chicken, canned, boneless, 3 oz.   170
  Turkey, roasted, skinned:
    Dark meat, 2½ by 1⅝ by ¼ in piece,
      4 pieces   175
    Light meat, 4 by 2 by ¼ in. piece, 2 pieces 150
    Light and dark meat, chopped or diced,
      1 cup   265

Fruits and Fruit Products

Apples:
  2¾-in. diam., 1   80
  3¼-in. diam., 1   125
Apple juice, 1 cup   120
Applesauce:
  Sweetened, 1 cup   230
  Unsweetened, 1 cup   100
Apricots:
  Fresh, 3   55
  Canned in heavy syrup, 1 cup   220
Apricot nectar, canned, 1 cup   145

Avocados (10 oz.), 1	370
Banana (2.6 per lb.), 1	100
Blackberries, 1 cup	85
Blueberries, 1 cup	90
Cherries:	
Sour, 1 cup	105
Sweet, 10 cherries	45
Cranberry juice cocktail, sweetened, 1 cup	165
Cranberry sauce, 1 cup	405
Dates, whole, 10	220
Fruit cocktail, canned in heavy syrup, 1 cup	195
Grapefruit:	
Fresh, medium:	
Pink or red, ½	50
White, ½	45
Grapefruit juice, 1 cup	95
Grapes:	
Thompson Seedless, 10	35
Tokay and Emperor, seeded types, 10	40
Grape juice:	
Canned or bottled, 1 cup	165
Frozen concentrate, sweetened, diluted with	
3 parts water by volume, 1 cup	135
Lemon, 1	20
Lemon juice, fresh, 1 cup	60
Lemonade concentrate, frozen, diluted with	4
4 1/3 parts water by volume, 1 cup	105
Limeade concentrate, frozen, diluted with 4 1/3	
parts water by volume, 1 cup	100
Lime juice, fresh, 1 cup	65
Muskmelons:	
Cantaloup, ½	80
Honeydew, 1/10	50
Oranges, whole, 2⅝-in. diam., 1	65
Orange juice:	
Canned, unsweetened, 1 cup	110
Frozen concentrate, diluted with 3 parts water	
by volume, 1 cup	120
Papayas, ½-in. cubes, 1 cup	55
Peaches:	

Fresh, 2½-in. diam., 1	40
Fresh, sliced, 1 cup	65
Canned in syrup, 1 cup	200
Canned in water, 1 cup	75
Pears:	
Bartlett, fresh, 2½-in. diam., 1	100
Bosc, fresh, 2½-in. diam., 1	85
D'Anjou, fresh, 3-in. diam., 1	120
Canned in heavy syrup, 1 cup	195
Pineapple:	
Fresh, diced, 1 cup	80
Canned in heavy syrup:	
Crushed, chunks, tidbits, 1 cup	190
Slice, large, 1 slice with 2¼ tbsp. liquid	80
Pineapple juice, unsweetened, canned, 1 cup	140
Plums:	
Fresh:	
Japanese and hybrid (2⅛-in. diam.), 1	30
Prune-type (1½-in. diam.), 1	20
Canned in heavy syrup, 3 with 2¾ tbsp. liquid	110
Prunes:	
Uncooked, 4 extra large or 5 large	110
Cooked, unsweetened with liquid, 1 cup	255
Raisins, seedless, 1 cup (not pressed down)	420
Raspberries, red, fresh, whole, 1 cup	70
Rhubarb, cooked, fresh, sugar added, 1 cup	380
Strawberries, raw, whole, 1 cup	55
Tangerine, fresh, 2⅜-in. diam., 1	40
Watermelon, 4 by 8 in. wedge	110

Grain Products

Bagel, 1	165
Barley, uncooked, 1 cup	700
Biscuits, baking powder, 2-in. diam., from home recipe, 1	105
Breads:	
Boston brown bread, canned, 1 3¼ by ½ in. slice	95
Raisin bread, enriched (18 slices per 1 lb. loaf), 1 slice	65

Rye bread:

American, 1 slice	60
Pumpernickel, 1 slice	80

White bread, enriched:

1 slice (18 per 1-lb. loaf)	70
1 slice (22 per 1-lb. loaf)	55
1 slice (24 per 1½-lb. loaf)	75
1 slice (28 per 1½-lb. loaf)	65
Whole-wheat bread (16 per 1 lb. loaf), 1 slice	65

Breakfast cereals:

Oatmeal or rolled oats, cooked, 1 cup	130

Ready-to-eat:

Bran flakes (40% bran), 1 cup	105
Corn flakes, 1 cup	95
Rice, puffed, 1 cup	60
Wheat, shredded, 1 oblong biscuit or ½ cup spoon-size	90

Cakes made from cake mixes:

Angelfood, 1/12 of cake	135
Devil's food, 2-layer with chocolate icing, 1/16 of cake	235
White, 2-layer with chocolate icing, 1/16 of cake	250
Fruitcake, dark, 1/30 of 1 lb. loaf	55
Pound, 1/17 of loaf	160
Spongecake, 1/12 of cake	195

Cookies:

Brownies with nuts, from home recipe, 1¾ x 1¾ x ⅞ in., 1	95
Chocolate chip, from home recipe, 2 1/3-in. diam., 4	205
Fig bars, rectangular, 4	200
Oatmeal with raisins, 2⅝-in. diam., ¼ in. thick, 4	235
Sandwich type (chocolate or vanilla), 4	200
Crackers, saltines, 4	50

Doughnuts:

Cake type, plain, 1	100
Yeast-leavened, glazed, 1	205
Macaroni, cooked, 1 cup	155

Noodles, cooked, 1 cup	200
Pancakes, from home recipe, 4-in. diam., 1	60
Pies:	
Apple, 1/7 of pie	345
Banana cream, 1/7 of pie	285
Blueberry, 1/7 of pie	325
Cherry, 1/7 of pie	350
Custard, 1/7 of pie	285
Pecan, 1/7 of pie	495
Pumpkin, 1/7 of pie	275
Pizza (cheese), ⅛ of 12-in. diam.	145
Popcorn, popped:	
Without oil, large kernel, 1 cup	25
With oil, 1 cup	40
Pretzels:	
Dutch, twisted, 2¾ by 2⅝ in., 1	60
Stick, 2¼-in. long, 10	10
Rice, white, cooked, 1 cup	225
Spaghetti, cooked, 1 cup	155
Waffle, from home recipe, 7-in. diam., 1	210

Legumes (dry), Nuts, Seeds, Related Products

Almonds, chopped, 1 cup	775
Beans:	
Cooked, drained:	
Great Northern, 1 cup	210
Pea (navy), 1 cup	225
Lima, 1 cup	260
Canned, red kidney, solids and liquid, 1 cup	230
Cashew nuts, roasted in oil, 1 cup	785
Peanut butter, 1 tbsp.	95
Peas, split, dry, cooked, 1 cup	230
Walnuts, Persian or English, 1 cup chopped	780

Sugars and Sweets

Candy:	
Caramels, plain or chocolate, 1 oz.	115
Chocolate, milk, plain, 1 oz.	145
Hard, 1 oz.	110

Honey, 1 tbsp.	65
Jams or preserves, 1 tbsp.	55
Jellies, 1 tbsp.	50
Syrups, table blends, chiefly corn, light and dark, 1 tbsp.	60
Sugars:	
Brown, 1 cup (packed)	820
White:	
Granulated, 1 cup	770
Granulated, 1 tbsp.	45
Powdered, sifted, 1 cup	385

Vegetable and Vegetable Products

Asparagus, cooked fresh, 1 cup	30
Beans:	
Lima, thick-seeded types, cooked, 1 cup	170
Snap:	
Green, cooked and drained, 1 cup	30
Yellow or wax, cooked and drained, 1 cup	30
Beets, peeled, diced or sliced, 1 cup	55
Broccoli, cooked and drained, 1 cup	40
Brussels sprouts, cooked, 1 cup	55
Cabbage:	
Raw, coarsely shredded or sliced, 1 cup	15
Cooked, drained, 1 cup	30
Carrots:	
Raw, 7½ by 1⅛ in., 1	30
Cooked, drained, 1 cup	50
Cauliflower, cooked, 1 cup	30
Celery, 1 stalk (8 by 1½ in.)	5
Corn, sweet:	
Ear, 5 in. long, 1	120
Canned, drained, 1 cup	140
Cucumber slices, ⅛ in. thick, 6½ large or 9 small pieces	5
Lettuce:	
Crisphead, as Iceberg, 6-in. diam., 1 head	70
Pieces, chopped or shredded, 1 cup	5
Mushrooms, raw, sliced or chopped, 1 cup	20

Onions, chopped, 1 cup	65
Peas, green	
Canned, whole, drained, 1 cup	150
Peppers, sweet, 1 pod	15
Potatoes, cooked:	
Baked, peeled after baking (about 2 per lb. raw), 1	145
Boiled (about 3 per lb. raw), peeled before boiling, 1	90
French-fried, 2 to 3½-in. long strip, 10	135
Potato chips, 10	115
Pumpkin, canned, 1 cup	80
Radishes, 4	5
Sauerkraut, 1 cup	40
Spinach, cooked, 1 cup	40
Squash, cooked:	
Summer (all varieties), diced, 1 cup	30
Winter (all varieties), mashed, 1 cup	130
Sweet potatoes (about 2½ per lb.), cooked, 1	160
Tomatoes:	
Raw, 2 3/5-in. diam., 1 tomato	25
Canned, 1 cup solids and liquid	50
Tomato catsup, 1 tbsp.	15
Tomato juice, 1 cup	45

Miscellaneous Items

Beverages, alcoholic:	
Beer, 12 fl. oz.	150
Gin, rum, vodka, whisky:	
80-proof, 1½-fl. oz. jigger	95
86-proof, 1½-fl. oz. jigger	105
90-proof, 1½-fl. oz. jigger	110
Wines:	
Dessert, 3½-fl. oz. glass	140
Table, 3½-fl. oz. glass	85
Beverages, carbonated, sweetened, nonalcoholic:	
Cola type, 12 fl. oz.	145
Fruit-flavored sodas, 12 fl. oz.	170

Olives:

Green, 4 medium or 3 extra large	15
Ripe, Mission, 3 small or 2 large	15

Soups, canned, condensed:

Prepared with equal volume of milk:

Cream of chicken, 1 cup	180
Cream of mushroom, 1 cup	215
Tomato, 1 cup	175

Prepared with equal volume of water:

Cream of chicken, 1 cup	95
Cream of mushroom, 1 cup	135
Tomato, 1 cup	90
Vegetarian, 1 cup	80

Equivalents by Volume

Level measure	*Equivalent*
1 gallon (3.786 liters; 8,786 milliliters)	4 quarts
1 quart (0.946 liter; 946 milliliters)	4 cups
1 cup (237 milliliters) 16 tablespoons	8 fluid ounces ½ pint
2 tablespoons (30 milliliters)	1 fluid ounce
1 tablespoon (15 milliliters)	3 teaspoons
1 pound regular butter or margarine	4 sticks 2 cups
1 pound whipped butter or margarine	6 sticks two 8-ounce containers 3 cups

Food Exchange Lists

Calorie-Free Foods

The following foods, seasonings, and beverages either have negligible calories or no calories at all. They may be used freely in reasonable amounts and do not have to be recorded on the food diary.

All raw vegetables from the vegetable exchange list	Mustard
	Onion flakes
Bouillon	Pickles (dill, unsweetened)
Broths, clear (no fat)	Pickles (sour)
Coffee	Rennet tablets
Cranberries (unsweetened)	Rhubarb (unsweetened)
Garlic	Saccharin
Gelatin (unflavored)	Soy sauce
Herbs	Spices
Horseradish	Tea
Lemon juice	Vinegar
Lime juice	

Meat Exchange List

Each meat exchange supplies approximately *75 calories* of energy. The lean meats will average somewhat less than this amount and the fat meats somewhat more. Always weigh meat after cooking.

List 1. The following are *lean* meats and *low-fat* cheeses, and increased use of these is encouraged:

Exchange	Amount to Use for 1 Exchange
Meat and poultry Chicken, game meats, liver and other organ meats, pheasant, rabbit, turkey, veal	1 ounce
Fish Bass, cod, flounder, haddock, halibut, lobster, salmon, trout, etc.	1 ounce
Crab, lobster, salmon, tuna	¼ cup (loosely packed)
Clams, oysters, scallops, shrimp	3-5 medium
Cheese Cottage cheese	1/3 cup
Skimmed or partially skimmed milk	1 1-inch cube or ounce

List 2. The following meat exchanges contain *more fat*; these should be used more sparingly.

Meat and poultry Beef, duck, goose, ham, lamb, pork	1 ounce
Eggs	1 egg
Cheese American (processed), cheddar, Edam, Swiss, etc.	1 slice (4 x 4 x ⅛ inches) or 1 1-inch cube or 1 ounce
Peanut butter	1 tablespoon
Cold cuts—bologna, salami, etc.	1 slice (4½ x 4½ x ⅛ inches)
Frankfurters (8-9 per lb.)	1 small
Sausage	1 small link

Bread Exchange List

Each bread exchange supplies approximately *70 calories* of energy. Soups and high-carbohydrate vegetables have been included on the cereal exchange list.

Exchange	Amount to Use for 1 Exchange
Breads and rolls	
Bagel	½
Bread dressing or stuffing	2 tablespoons
Hamburger, hot dog bun (large)	½ bun
Matzos	1 6-inch diameter
White, whole-wheat, rye	1 slice (1 ounce)
Quick breads	
Biscuit, roll, muffin	1 2-inch diameter
Corn bread	1 piece 1½-inch cube
Doughnut, plain	1 small
English muffin	½
Pancake	1 4-inch diameter cake
Waffle	1 4-inch diameter waffle
Crackers	
Graham	2 crackers, 2½-inches square
Oyster	½ cup
Round	5 crackers, 2-inches diameter
Rye	2 double crackers
Saltines	5 crackers, 2-inches square
Soda	3 crackers, 2½-inches square
Cereals	
Cooked: grits, oats, rice, wheat	½ cup
Ready-to-eat: flake and puff types	1 ounce
Flour	2½ tablespoons
Vegetables and soups	
Baked beans in sauce (no pork)	¼ cup
Corn	1 small ear or ½ cup kernels
Dried beans, lentils, peas (cooked)	½ cup
Parsnips	½ cup
Popcorn (no butter)	3 cups

Potatoes	1 small or ½ cup mashed
Potatoes, sweet or yams	¼ cup
Soup, meat or vegetable	1 serving (3 per can)
Soup, cream, pea, or bean	½ serving (3 per can)

Milk Exchange List

Each milk exchange supplies approximately *85 calories* of energy. Skimmed or partially skimmed milk should be used.

Exchange	Amount to Use for 1 Exchange
Buttermilk (skimmed)	1 cup (8 ounces)
Cottage cheese (creamed)	1/3 cup
Cottage cheese (plain)	½ cup
Evaporated milk	¼ cup
Evaporated milk (skimmed)	½ cup
Ice milk	1/3 cup
Nonfat dried milk powder	¼ cup
Partially skimmed milk	¾ cup
Skimmed milk	1 cup
Yogurt, plain (made from partially skimmed milk)	¾ cup
Yogurt, plain (made from skimmed milk)	1 cup

Vegetable Exchange List

Three vegetable exchanges (two from the first list and one from the second) supply approximately *50 calories*.

List 1. The following vegetables provide negligible calories. In raw form they may be eaten as desired in reasonable amounts and do not need to be recorded on the daily food plan. When cooked, limit serving portions to ½ to 1 cup and record as one vegetable exchange.

Asparagus

Bamboo shoots

Broccoli

Brussels sprouts

Cabbage

Cauliflower

Celery

Cucumber

Eggplant

Endive

Green beans

Green onions

Greens
  Beet greens
  Chard
  Collards
  Dandelion greens

Kale

Mustard greens

Spinach

Turnip greens

Kohlrabi

Lettuce

Mushrooms

Okra

Peppers

Radishes

Sauerkraut

Summer squash

Tomatoes

Tomato Juice

Watercress

List 2. The following vegetables are slightly higher in calories. When cooked, average one serving of these vegetables daily, but limit serving portions to ½ cup and count as one vegetable exchange. When used in the raw form, it is not necessary to record these as a vegetable exchange on your food diary, but use these raw vegetables less frequently that those from List 1.

Artichokes

Beets

Carrots

Onions

Peas

Pea pods

Pumpkin

Rutabagas

Turnips

Winter squash

Fruit Exchange List

Each fruit exchange provides approximately *40 calories* of energy. Fruits may be fresh, dried, cooked, canned, or frozen as long as *no sugar* is added. Those in bold type are especially rich in vitamin C. At least one vitamin C-rich fruit should be eaten daily.

Exchange	Amount to Use for 1 Exchange
Apple	1 small or ½ medium
Apple juice	½ cup
Applesauce	½ cup
Apricots	2
Apricots, dried	4 halves
Banana	½ small
Blackberries	1 cup
Blueberries	1 cup
Cantaloupe	¼ small
Cherries	12
Figs, fresh	2
Grapes	12
Grape juice	¼ cup
Grapefruit	½ small
Grapefruit juice	½ cup
Guava	1
Honeydew melon	⅛
Mango	½ small
Orange	1 small
Orange juice	½ cup
Papaya	½ small
Peach	1
Pear	1 small
Pineapple	½ cup
Pineapple juice	½ cup
Plums	2
Raisins	2 tablespoons

Raspberries	1 cup
Strawberries	1 cup
Watermelon	1 cup

Miscellaneous Foods Exchange List

These foods and beverages provide concentrated sources of calories.

List 1 (Fats). Each of these provides approximately *40 calories* per exchange.

Exchange	Amount to Use for 1 Exchange
Avocado	⅛ 4-inch diameter
Bacon, crisp	1 slice
Butter or margarine	1 teaspoon
Cream, light	2 tablespoons
Cream, heavy or sour	1 tablespoon
Cream cheese	1 tablespoon
French dressing	1 tablespoon
Mayonnaise	1 teaspoon
Nuts	6 small
Oil or cooking fat	1 teaspoon
Olives	5 small

List 2 (Sweets). The following sweets provide approximately *40 calories* per exchange.

Exchange	Amount to Use for 1 Exchange
Cocoa (sweetened)	1 level tablespoon or 1 heaping teaspoon
Hard candy (small) or caramel	1

Sugar, syrup, honey, jam, jelly	1 level tablespoon or 1 heaping teaspoon

List 3 (Desserts and beverages). These foods, in the amounts specified, supply approximately *80 calories* and *must be counted as 2 miscellaneous* food exchanges.

Exchange	**Amount to Use for 2 Exchanges**
Desserts	
Cake: sponge, angel food, made with enriched flour	1 piece, 2 x 2 x 1 inches
Jello	1 serving (5 per package)
Sherbet	1/3 cup
Any dessert, if 1 serving portion is no more than 80 calories	
Beverages	
Beer	6 ounces
Light Beer	12 ounces
Carbonated beverages	6 ounces
Gin, rum, whiskey *	1 ounce
Liqueur (creme de menthe, etc.)	1 ounce
Wine (red, sweet)	2 ounces
Wine (light, dry)	3 ounces

* Note that one jigger is 1½ ounces and would be counted as 3 miscellaneous food exchanges.